Aids to Medicine for Nurses

Aids to Medicine for Nurses

J.L. Burton
B.Sc., M.D., M.R.C.P.
Consultant Senior Lecturer in Dermatology,
Bristol Royal Infirmary

CHURCHILL LIVINGSTONE
EDINBURGH LONDON AND NEW YORK 1976

CHURCHILL LIVINGSTONE
Medical Division of Longman Group Limited

Distributed in the United States of America by
Longman Inc., 72 Fifth Avenue, New York,
N.Y. 10011 and by associated companies,
branches and representatives throughout
the world.

© Longman Group Limited, 1976

All rights reserved. No part of this publication may be reproduced, stored in a retrieval system, or transmitted in any form or by any means, electronic, mechanical, photocopying, recording or otherwise, without the prior permission of the publishers (Churchill Livingstone, 23 Ravelston Terrace, Edinburgh).

First published 1976

ISBN 0 443 01387 X

Printed in Great Britain

Preface

This little book aims to help nurses revising for their medical examinations. Many examiners condemn learning by rote, but I believe that the use of factual lists can greatly facilitate revision. Such lists, if used sensibly in conjunction with larger textbooks throughout the course, provide a useful skeleton for answering examination questions, and they encourage an orderly approach to the subject.

Such a small book cannot be comprehensive, but I have tried to cover the subjects which occur most frequently in final examination papers in Medical Nursing, and to pay particular attention to those subjects which nurses find most difficult. In each chapter I have given a brief review of the important anatomy and physiology of a particular system, followed by a summary of the causes, clinical features, complications and treatment of the common diseases which occur in that system. Ward organization and practical nursing procedures have not been included, but I have included sections on the testing of urine, sputum and faeces, and there is also a chapter on the use of common drugs.

I should like to thank my nursing colleagues in the School of Nursing, in the Bristol Health District, who have helped me enormously in writing this book by making many useful suggestions and by reading and correcting the manuscript.

1976   J.L.B.

Contents

	Page
Preface	v
Cardiovascular system	1
Respiratory system	19
Digestive system	35
Nervous system	52
Urinary system	67
Reproduction	80
Endocrinology	85
Haematology	94
Dermatology	106
Bones and joints	112
Drugs	119
Index	127

Cardiovascular system

The heart is a muscle pump whose function is to perfuse the tissues with blood by contracting rhythmically. In a resting adult the heart expels about 5 litres of blood each minute (*cardiac output*)
    The *pericardium* is a two-layered sac which encloses the heart
    The *myocardium* is the heart muscle
    The *endocardium* lines the 4 heart chambers and covers the 4 heart valves

The 4 chambers are: The 4 valves are:

1. The R. and L. atria   1. The aortic and pulmonary valves
2. The R. and L. ventricles   2. The mitral and tricuspid valves

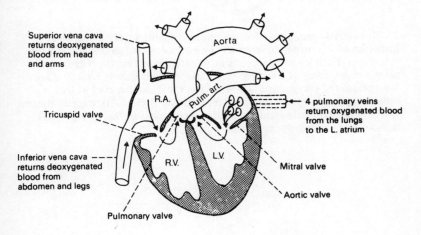

THE CARDIAC CYCLE

Atrial contraction (*atrial systole*) squeezes blood into the ventricles while they are relaxed (*ventricular diastole*). The ventricles then contract (*ventricular systole*) to expel blood into the aorta and R. and L. pulmonary arteries while the atria relax (*atrial diastole*) and refill with blood from the superior and inferior venae cavae and pulmonary veins.

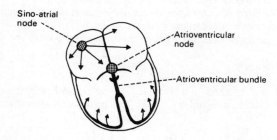

This regular sequence of contraction is maintained by electrical impulses which originate from the *sino-atrial node* (*pacemaker*) in the R. atrium. Each impulse spreads in all directions over both atria, and after a short delay at the *atrioventricular node* it travels rapidly down the specialized conducting tissue (*atrioventricular bundle*) in the interventricular septum to stimulate both ventricles. After each impulse the conducting tissue requires a short rest period (*refractory period*) before another impulse can pass.

THE ARTERIAL PULSE
Observe
1. Rate
2. Rhythm
3. Character

1. *RATE*
Normal: Resting adult   60–85 beats/min
         Resting child   80–100 beats/min
         Newborn infant   100–130 beats/min

Causes of rapid pulse (tachycardia)
1. Exercise or emotion
2. Fever
3. Bleeding
4. Thyrotoxicosis
5. Heart disease e.g. cardiac failure
6. Cardiac arrhythmia

Causes of slow pulse (bradycardia)
1. Physical training
2. Myxoedema
3. Raised intra-cranial pressure
4. Drugs e.g. digitalis
5. Heart block

Pulse deficit. If some ventricular contractions fail to produce a radial pulse beat the *apex rate* (felt or heard at the heart apex) will exceed the rate at the wrist. This is called a 'pulse deficit'

Causes of a pulse deficit
1. Extrasystoles
2. Atrial fibrillation

2. RHYTHM

Common causes of an irregular pulse
1. Sinus arrhythmia
2. Extrasystoles
3. Atrial fibrillation

1. Sinus arrhythmia
A physiological increase in pulse rate during inspiration. Common in children and during convalescence

2. Extrasystole (ectopic beat)
An extrasystole is a premature beat due to a cardiac impulse arising at an abnormal (ectopic) site in the heart. The pulse beat felt at the wrist is usually weak. This is followed by a *compensatory pause* and the next beat is unusually forceful. Extrasystoles are common and may not be dangerous

Causes of extrasystoles
- i Fatigue
- ii Excessive smoking or ingestion of alcohol or coffee
- iii Heart disease e.g. mitral stenosis or myocardial ischaemia
- iv Drugs e.g. digitalis
- v Thyrotoxicosis

3. Atrial fibrillation
Very rapid uncoordinated contractions of muscle bundles occur all over the atria, and the ventricles are stimulated rapidly and irregularly. The pulse rate is about 100–180 beats/min unless controlled by digitalis

Causes of atrial fibrillation
- i Rheumatic heart disease (e.g. mitral stenosis)
- ii Myocardial ischaemia
- iii Thyrotoxicosis

3. CHARACTER (Quality)

i Volume
A full pulse may be due to a hyperdynamic circulation e.g. fever, pregnancy, thyrotoxicosis

A weak pulse may be due to dehydration, blood loss, myocardial infarction or 'shock'

ii Tension
This depends on the blood pressure (high BP = hypertension). Tension cannot be accurately assessed by palpation and a sphygomomanometer should be used

iii Pulse wave
Variations in the pulse wave may be helpful in diagnosis

In aortic *incompetence* the pulse beat has a 'slapping' quality (*collapsing pulse*)

In aortic *stenosis* the pulse beat is sustained (*plateau pulse*)

iv State of the artery
Normal arteries are soft and elastic

Arteriosclerotic arteries are hard and rigid

JUGULAR VENOUS PULSE (J.V.P.)

The pressure in the jugular veins can be estimated by inspecting the neck in the recumbent patient with the head and shoulders raised $30°$ from the horizontal. The pressure is increased in heart failure and obstruction of the superior vena cava. The shape of the venous pulse wave may be abnormal in tricuspid valve disease and in constrictive pericarditis.

GENERAL SYMPTOMS OF HEART DISEASE

1. **Dyspnoea**, especially on exertion
   Orthopnoea is a later stage in which breathlessness forces the patient to remain sitting up
   Paroxysmal nocturnal dyspnoea is characterized by the sudden onset of dyspnoea and wheezing, with a sense of suffocation. It usually occurs at night, and is due to pulmonary congestion with the patient lying flat
2. **Palpitation** (awareness of the heart beat) occurs in normal subjects and in patients with heart disease
3. **Chest pain.** Very variable, but often precipitated by exertion or a heavy meal, and spreads into the neck or arms
4. **Oedema** of the most dependent parts (usually ankles or sacrum)
5. **Cerebral symptoms** due to impaired oxygenation of the brain. These include insomnia and memory loss
6. **Digestive disturbance** due to gastro-intestinal congestion

BLOOD PRESSURE

The BP should be measured with the patient resting and relaxed. It rises with age but normal values in adults are:
   Systolic   =   100 to 140 mm Hg
   Diastolic =   60 to 90 mm Hg
   Pulse pressure (systolic minus diastolic) = 30 to 60 mm Hg
Old people with arteriosclerosis often have a raised systolic pressure and a normal diastolic pressure. This is of little significance, but increased diastolic pressure is always important

HYPOTENSION

Low systolic BP

Causes

1. Vasovagal attack ('fainting')
2. Systemic infections e.g. 'flu, enteric fever
3. Myocardial infarction
4. Dehydration or bleeding
5. Hypoadrenalism

HYPERTENSION
BP more than 150/90

Causes
1. Essential hypertension (cause unknown)
2. Secondary
    - *i* Renal disease e.g. nephritis or renal ischaemia
    - *ii* Rarely coarctation of aorta, phaeochromocytoma, Cushing's disease etc.

Malignant hypertension is severe hypertension characterized by a diastolic pressure over 140 mm Hg, retinal changes (papilloedema and haemorrhages) and progressive renal failure

Clinical features of hypertension
1. May be no symptoms
2. 'Fullness' in the head, throbbing headache, giddiness
3. Left ventricular failure, palpitations
4. Arterial degeneration
5. Retinopathy
6. Albuminuria and renal failure
7. Cerebral thrombosis or haemorrhage

Treatment of hypertension
1. Weight reduction, avoidance of stress and strain, stopping smoking
2. Drugs—for mild hypertension (diastolic 90 to 110 mm Hg) a sedative or a regular diuretic such as *chlorothiazide* may be sufficient. Drugs for moderate or severe hypertension include *guanethidine, methyldopa* and *bethanidine.* Treatment is for life, and regular BP checks are required
   Pentolinium may be injected to reduce BP rapidly in an emergency

CARDIAC ARRHYTHMIAS
1. **Extrasystoles** (p. 4)
2. **Atrial fibrillation** (p. 4)
3. **Atrial flutter**

    An uncommon arrhythmia due to heart disease. The pulse rate is rapid and regular but may vary due to changes in the degree of heart block (q.v.)

4. **Paroxysmal tachycardia**

    Rapid heart-beats, often of sudden onset, due to regular discharge of impulses from an ectopic focus in the atria, atrioventricular node or ventricles. The attacks cause palpitations and usually stop suddenly after a few seconds, minutes or days

HEART BLOCK

This refers to impairment of the conduction of the impulses through the AV node and the atrio-ventricular bundle. Mild degrees may be seen only on an electrocardiogram, but in more severe degrees there is bradycardia (about 36 beats/min) with the atria and ventricles contracting independently of each other

Stokes-Adams attacks are periods of unconsciousness from cerebral anoxia due to transient cardiac arrest as a result of unstable heart block. The patient is very pale during the attack but becomes flushed as consciousness returns

VALVULAR DISEASE
CAUSES
1. Congenital (p. 9)
2. Rheumatic heart disease (p. 11)
3. Infective endocarditis (p. 12)
4. Syphilis (p. 12)

CONGENITAL HEART DISEASE
Classified into 2 groups, cyanotic and acyanotic

1. **Cyanotic**

   Fallot's tetralogy, the commonest example, consists of:

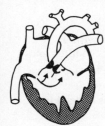

   1. Pulmonary stenosis
   2. Ventricular septal defect
   3. Over-riding aorta, which lies over both ventricles
   4. R. ventricular hypertrophy

   Clinical features of Fallot's tetralogy:
   1. Cyanosis and polycythaemia
   2. Dyspnoea on exertion (relieved by squatting)
   3. Clubbing of fingers
   4. Impaired growth
   5. Systolic heart murmur

2. **Acyanotic** (i.e. without cyanosis)

   Coarctation of the aorta

   Narrowing of the aorta, usually just below the L subclavian artery. The BP is usually raised in the head and arms, but the femoral pulses are delayed and diminished. The prognosis is variable

   Persistent ductus arteriosus

   This duct should close at, or soon after birth, but if it persists, the shunt from the aorta to the pulmonary artery causes increased pulmonary blood flow and a murmur. These patients may develop cardiac failure or subacute bacterial endocarditis (p. 12)

   Pulmonary stenosis

   Mild cases may have no symptoms but severe cases develop cardiac failure before middle life

(contd.)

Atrial septal defect

Blood from the L. atrium passes through the hole into the R. atrium and thus re-enters the pulmonary circulation. There may be few symptoms until middle age, when cardiac failure develops

Ventricular septal defect

A small defect will produce a murmur without symptoms, but a large defect will allow so much blood to enter the R. ventricle from the L. ventricle that the pulmonary circulation becomes overloaded and pulmonary hypertension develops.

'Innocent' murmurs

The majority of systolic murmurs are harmless and may be disregarded. These 'innocent' murmurs are common in children and in the elderly

RHEUMATIC FEVER

Aetiology. Probably an allergic reaction to infection with a *haemolytic Streptococcus* (usually tonsillitis). It affects children and young adults, but is now uncommon in Britain

Clinical features

1. Fever and 'flitting' joint pains, especially in knees and ankles
2. Cardiac involvement
   - *i* Tachycardia
   - *ii* Cardiac murmurs
   - *iii* Cardiac enlargement or failure
   - *iv* Pericarditis
3. Rash or subcutaneous nodules

Treatment

1. Rest, with support for the joints and a high fluid intake
2. Salicylates such as aspirin in high dosage
   Steroid therapy is sometimes used for carditis
3. Penicillin may be used to eradicate the Streptococcus and long-term penicillin prevents further attacks

Complete rest must be enforced for many weeks, until all signs of active disease have gone and the plasma viscosity or ESR is normal

Rheumatic chorea

This is a similar allergic process affecting the brain. Affected children become restless and fidgety, with involuntary movements and grimaces. The disease lasts about 2 months, but some cases develop rheumatic heart disease

RHEUMATIC HEART DISEASE

Rheumatic fever causes endocarditis with small 'vegetations' (fibrin, platelets and leucocytes) on the valves. These are replaced by fibrous scar tissue which gradually contracts and deforms the valve so it either becomes narrowed (*stenosis*) or fails to close properly (*incompetence*). There is usually a latent period of 15—20 years before symptoms such as dyspnoea appear. The mitral and aortic valves are most commonly affected.

Mitral stenosis

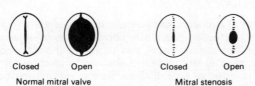

Mitral stenosis obstructs the flow from L. atrium to L. ventricle and this causes a rise in pressure in the L. atrium. At first the heart compensates by enlargement of the atrium and hypertrophy of its walls, but later the pressure in the pulmonary circulation rises. The resulting pulmonary congestion causes dyspnoea and the patient may develop attacks of acute pulmonary oedema. Eventually R. ventricular failure occurs.

Clinical features
1. Pulmonary congestion
    * *i* Progressive exertional dyspnoea
    * *ii* Orthopnoea (dyspnoea when lying flat)
    * *iii* Paroxysmal nocturnal dyspnoea ('cardiac asthma')
    * *iv* Cough and haemoptysis
2. Loud first heart sound with a soft diastolic murmur
3. Often a thin face with purple cheeks ('malar flush')

Complications
1. Atrial fibrillation
2. Acute pulmonary oedema
3. R. ventricular failure
4. Thrombus in L. atrium and systemic emboli (e.g. cerebral)
5. Subacute bacterial endocarditis
6. Recurrent bronchitis

Treatment
1. Treatment of cardiac failure (p. 13)
2. Mitral valvotomy or valve replacement

Mitral incompetence

This may be due to rheumatic heart disease or it may be secondary to L. ventricular failure and dilatation. There is a loud systolic murmur at the apex

Aortic stenosis

This causes a harsh systolic murmur over the aorta but there may be few symptoms for many years. Eventually L. ventricular failure, angina or syncope ('black-outs') may result

INFECTIVE ENDOCARDITIS

Acute bacterial endocarditis is usually due to bacteria (e.g. Staphylococci) or fungi affecting previously normal valves in seriously ill patients. Large 'vegetations' cause destruction of the affected valves with murmurs, cardiac failure, septicaemia and widespread infarcts and abscesses due to infected emboli. Treatment is with antibiotics in large doses, but the disease is often fatal

Subacute bacterial endocarditis (SABE) is a less severe disease due to *Streptococcus viridans* which attacks previously damaged valves

Clinical features of SABE
1. Heart murmur
2. Fever, weight loss, anaemia
3. Small haemorrhages in the skin (purpura) or nails ('splinter haemorrhages')
4. Finger clubbing
5. Enlarged spleen (splenomegaly)

Treatment

Penicillin in large doses for at least six weeks. To prevent SABE, patients known to have cardiac damage should receive penicillin 'cover' for dental extractions

SYPHILIS

Tertiary syphilis may cause *aortic incompetence* or *aortic aneurysm*

CARDIAC FAILURE

Heart failure is the inability of the heart to maintain the normal circulation. Either the L. side or the R. side of the heart may fail first, but eventually both sides will be involved

L. VENTRICULAR FAILURE

Causes
1. Myocardial ischaemia
2. Hypertension
3. Aortic stenosis or incompetence

Clinical features
1. Pulmonary congestion or pulmonary oedema
2. Tachycardia
3. Cardiac enlargement
4. Cyanosis

R. VENTRICULAR FAILURE

Causes
1. Following L. ventricular failure
2. Mitral stenosis
3. Pulmonary disease e.g. chronic bronchitis
4. Congenital heart disease

Clinical features
1. Tiredness and weakness
2. Digestive disturbances (due to gastro-intestinal congestion)
3. Oedema of dependent parts (ankles, sacrum)
4. Increased jugular venous pressure
5. Large tender liver, often with ascites

Treatment of cardiac failure

Mild cases may be controlled by increased rest, reduction of obesity, avoidance of physical and mental stress, and a regular diuretic (p. 119) with potassium

Moderate cases may need digitalis and a low-salt diet in addition

Severe cases may need bed rest with the legs dependent (cardiac bed), high concentration oxygen therapy, and i.v. aminophylline, frusemide and morphine

The nurse should watch for evidence of digitalis toxicity (p. 119)

PULMONARY OEDEMA

Causes
1. Left atrial or ventricular failure
2. Severe pneumonia
3. Excess of intra-venous fluid
4. Inhalation of irritant gas e.g. chlorine

Clinical features

The patient is orthopnoeic and distressed, usually cyanosed, and coughing up large quantities of white or pink frothy sputum. The pulse is rapid and in severe cases the BP falls and 'shock' ensues

Treatment
1. High concentration oxygen therapy with patient sitting up with legs dependent
2. Intravenous morphine, frusemide and aminophylline
3. Digitalis

MYOCARDIAL ISCHAEMIA

The R. and L. coronary arteries arise from the aorta and supply the myocardium. Narrowing of the lumen of these arteries by atheroma or thrombosis leads to myocardial ischaemia which may produce angina or infarction

Factors predisposing to coronary artery disease
1. Increased blood lipids (? due to high intake of animal fat or sucrose)
2. Hypertension
3. Cigarette smoking
4. Lack of exercise and obesity
5. Diabetes mellitus
6. Family history of myocardial infarction

ANGINA PECTORIS

Crushing substernal pain, usually provoked by effort or emotion and relieved by rest. It may radiate into the neck or down the L. arm or both arms. ECG usually shows changes of myocardial ischaemia. Treatment is with trinitrin (chewed slowly) or a beta-blocker (p. 120) and moderation of the patient's way of life

MYOCARDIAL INFARCTION

A plaque of atheroma or a clot in a branch of a coronary artery (*coronary thrombosis*) may occlude the vessel completely and cause necrosis (*infarction*) of an area of the myocardium

Clinical features
1. Sudden angina, which may occur at rest, and persists for hours
2. May be dyspnoea, intense anxiety, syncope or vomiting
3. Pallor or cyanosis, sweating, tachycardia, hypotension

Common complications
1. L. ventricular failure
2. Cardiac arrhythmia or heart block
3. Cardiac arrest
4. 'Shock'
5. Pericarditis
6. Pulmonary embolism (from leg vein thrombosis)
7. Systemic embolism from clot on the infarcted area
8. Rupture or aneurysm of the cardiac wall

Treatment
1. Admission to intensive care unit with constant ECG monitoring and facilities to deal with cardiac arrest
2. The patient should rest comfortably in bed and be spared undue movement and anxiety
3. Analgesics (e.g. diamorphine or pethidine) should be given as necessary
4. Cardiac failure is treated with high conc. oxygen and diuretics
5. Anticoagulants are sometimes used to prevent embolism
6. Drugs such as atropine, lignocaine or phenytoin may be needed to treat or prevent arrhythmias

COMMON CAUSES OF CHEST PAIN

1. Myocardial ischaemia e.g. coronary atheroma, severe anaemia
2. Pericarditis
3. Pleurisy
4. Pulmonary embolism
5. Oesophageal pain e.g. carcinoma, hiatus hernia
6. Pain from chest wall e.g. fractured rib, herpes zoster
7. Pain referred from the abdomen e.g. gastric ulcer or gallstones

CARDIAC ARREST

This is recognized by the fact that the patient is unconscious and has no pulse. The pupils may or may not be dilated. Since irreversible brain damage occurs within 2–3 minutes the nurse must call for help and start immediate resuscitation, as follows:
1. Make sure the patient is on a firm surface (e.g. floor or fracture boards)
2. Clear the airway (remove dentures and extend the neck)
3. Commence artificial respiration (mouth-to-mouth or Ambu bag, 15 breaths per minute) and external cardiac massage (60 compressions of the sternum per minute)

Remember to close the nostrils and support the jaw during artificial respiration. If resuscitation is effective the pulse should be palpable and the dilated pupils should contract. When help arrives the patient will be intubated and ventilated with oxygen. An i.v. infusion of drugs such as sodium bicarbonate, lignocaine and calcium chloride will be administered and defibrillating shocks will be applied.

Cardiac arrest is due either to cessation of ventricular activity (*cardiac asystole*) or to *ventricular fibrillation.* An ECG is needed to distinguish these two possibilities, but resuscitation must not be delayed to obtain records.

PERICARDITIS

Inflammation of the pericardium may be *dry* or associated with a fluid *effusion*

Causes
1. Myocardial infarction
2. 'Benign' pericarditis (usually viral)
3. Bacterial e.g. TB, pneumonia, septicaemia
4. Rheumatic fever
5. Severe uraemia

Clinical features of dry pericarditis
1. Substernal pain, often related to respiration
2. Cough, dyspnoea, pyrexia and tachycardia
3. Pericardial friction rub

Clinical features of pericardial effusion
1. Substernal discomfort and dyspnoea
2. Raised venous pressure
3. Large effusions may reduce the cardiac output

In *chronic constrictive pericarditis* the heart is enclosed by fibrous tissue (often calcified) due to previous TB. This impedes the normal filling of the heart and may need to be removed surgically

THROMBOSIS
A blood clot in the heart, arteries or veins
Common sites include:
1. Heart
    - *i* Left atrium, in mitral stenosis
    - *ii* Left ventricle, in myocardial infarction
2. Arteries
    - *i* Coronary
    - *ii* Cerebral
3. Veins
    - *i* Superficial varicose veins in the leg
    - *ii* Deep veins of the calf
    - *iii* Femoral or iliac veins e.g. in pregnancy
    - *iv* Haemorrhoids ('piles')

Predisposing factors
1. Damage to lining of the heart or blood-vessel e.g. atheroma
2. Slowing of blood-flow e.g. prolonged bed-rest
3. Increased blood coagulability e.g. oestrogen therapy

'Deep-vein thrombosis' (DVT) of the calf
Clinical features
1. Slight pyrexia
2. Pain and tenderness in the calf, worse on dorsiflexion of the foot
3. Oedema of the ankle
4. May be no symptoms until pulmonary embolism occurs

Prevention of DVT
1. Leg exercises, calf massage and early mobilisation
2. Avoidance of anything which impedes venous return from the legs
3. Anticoagulants

EMBOLISM

An *embolus* is a foreign body which is transported from one part of the circulatory system to another, where it becomes impacted. This process is called *embolism*. It cuts off the blood supply to the affected part, which usually produces an area of necrosis called an *infarct*.

Causes of embolism

1. Blood clot (thrombus) from heart or leg veins
2. Air entering veins during operation or due to injury
3. Fat from a fractured bone
4. Clumps of bacteria from heart valves in bacterial endocarditis

Pulmonary embolism occurs when an embolus from the venous circulation reaches the pulmonary arteries or one of their branches in the lungs

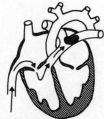

Clinical features depend on the size of the infarct. There may be chest pain, haemoptysis, dyspnoea or sudden death

Clot from
D.V.T. blocking
L. pulmonary artery

Cerebral embolism is usually due to an embolus from the *left* side of the heart. It produces sudden loss of function of a part of the brain, resulting, for example, in coma, paralysis or loss of speech.

Embolism of a limb artery causes a pale or blue limb which may be painful or numb. The pulse in the limb disappears and the limb feels cold to the touch. Unless the circulation is quickly re-established gangrene may result.

Phlebitis (inflammation of a vein). Often occurs in varicose veins, or at a site of injury or infection.

Superficial phlebitis causes pain and redness, and the vein can be felt as a tender cord. The inflammation may cause a clot to form (*thrombophlebitis*).

Respiratory system

The *upper respiratory tract* consists of:
1. The nose and paranasal air sinuses
2. The pharynx, larynx and trachea

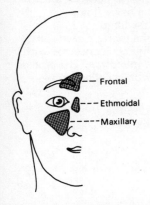

The paranasal air sinuses

The *frontal, ethmoidal* and *maxillary* sinuses are as shown. The *sphenoidal* sinuses lie behind the upper part of the nasal cavity

The *lower respiratory tract* consists of:
1. The bronchi, bronchioles and alveolar ducts
2. The alveoli (air cells) in the lung

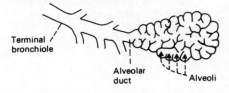

The alveoli are surrounded by the pulmonary capillaries

RESPIRATION

Respiration allows oxygen (O_2) to be taken up by the tissues and carbon dioxide (CO_2) to be eliminated from the body

External respiration refers to the absorption of O_2 from the air, and the elimination of CO_2 by the lungs. This exchange of gases occurs by diffusion across the alveolar membrane and the capillary endothelium. CO_2 elimination regulates the pH of the blood

Internal respiration refers to the gaseous exchange between the cells in the various body tissues and their surrounding tissue fluids

Ventilation (movement of air in and out of the lungs)

This is brought about by changes in size of the thoracic cavity, the lungs following these variations passively. The muscles concerned with inspiration are the *diaphragm* and the *external intercostals*. The process of breathing is controlled by the *respiratory centre,* a collection of neurones in the medulla of the brain

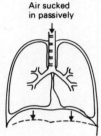

Air sucked in passively

The diaphragm is attached to the bottom of the thoracic cage and it flattens as it contracts

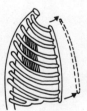

The external intercostals elevate the ribs and this pushes the sternum forward

RESPIRATORY RATE

The normal rate is about 12—20 per min in the adult and 40 per min in the infant

The normal respiration: pulse ratio is about 1:4

Causes of rapid respiration
1. Exertion, excitement or fever
2. Anoxaemia (decreased oxygen content of blood)
3. Pain associated with breathing e.g. pleurisy or peritonitis may cause rapid shallow respiration

Causes of slow respiration
Depression of respiratory centre e.g. terminal illness, head injury, barbiturate overdose

Dyspnoea (a feeling of breathlessness)

Causes
1. Pulmonary or cardiac disease
2. Obstruction to air entry into lungs
3. Acidosis (e.g. renal failure)
4. Psychological (e.g. anxiety)

RESPIRATORY RHYTHM

Inspiration and expiration should take an equal time
Prolonged *inspiration* occurs in laryngeal or tracheal obstruction (e.g. croup)
Prolonged *expiration* occurs in bronchial obstruction (e.g. asthma)

Cheyne-Stokes breathing. The depth of respiration increases progressively to a maximum, then diminishs to a period of apnoea (absent breathing) and the cycle is repeated

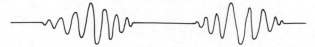

This is due to decreased sensitivity of the respiratory centre to CO_2

Common causes of Cheyne-Stokes breathing
1. Severe cardiac failure
2. Pneumonia
3. Barbiturate overdose
4. Cerebro-vascular accident
5. Head injury

'Air hunger' (Kussmaul's breathing) consists of very deep respirations due to stimulation of the respiratory centre by acidosis

Common causes of 'air hunger'
1. Terminal renal failure
2. Uncontrolled diabetes mellitus

Stertorous breathing is a noisy snoring type of respiration which occurs in unconscious patients

CHEST SHAPE

May be abnormal in:
1. **Lung disease**
    i *Fibrosis* (e.g. due to TB) may flatten the affected area
    ii *Emphysema* may produce a barrel-shaped chest
2. **Bone disease**
    i *Spinal kyphosis* (anterior bending) or *scoliosis* (lateral bending) may restrict lung movement
    ii *Rickets* may cause flattening of the rib cage due to bending of the soft ribs

CLUBBING

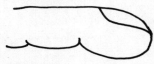

A bulbous enlargement of the terminal phalanges, with curved nails and filling-in of the angle at the nail base

Causes
1. Bronchial carcinoma
2. Chronic pulmonary suppuration
3. Bacterial endocarditis
4. Cyanotic congenital heart disease

COUGH AND SPUTUM
Types of cough, and their causes
1. *Dry* (without sputum)
    i Diseases of throat, larynx or trachea
    ii Early stages of pneumonia
    iii Psychological ('nervous' cough)
2. *Productive* (with sputum)
    i Bronchitis
    ii TB
    iii Pneumonia
    iv Bronchiectasis or lung abscess
3. *Spasmodic* (a series of explosive coughs)
    i Whooping cough
    ii 'Croup'
4. *'Brassy'* (characteristic noise due to pressure on the trachea)
    Aortic aneurysm

Types of sputum
1. *Mucoid* (clear or white)
    i Chronic bronchitis
    ii Asthma

   In asthma there may be sticky plugs ('casts' of the bronchial tree)
2. *Purulent* (yellow or green)

   May occur with any lung infection. In bronchiectasis and lung abscess the sputum is often copious and foul-smelling
3. *Haemoptysis* (blood-stained)
    i Pulmonary disease e.g. bronchial carcinoma, TB
    ii Cardiac disease e.g. mitral stenosis

   In lobar pneumonia the sputum may be rust-coloured
4. *Pink, frothy and copious*
   Pulmonary oedema

Microscopic examination of the sputum may reveal *bacteria* (e.g. in bronchitis, TB or pneumonia), *eosinophils* (in allergic asthma) or *malignant cells* (in bronchial carcinoma)

Culture of the sputum enables bacteria to be identified, and their sensitivity to various antibiotics to be tested

BRONCHITIS
Inflammation of the bronchial mucosa

ACUTE BRONCHITIS
Causes
1. Downward spread of upper respiratory infection e.g. coryza or sinusitis
2. Systemic viral infection e.g. measles or influenza
3. Irritant gases e.g. 'smog' or smoke

Clinical features
1. Pyrexia
2. Central chest soreness
3. Cough, with or without sputum
4. Dyspnoea and wheezing with cyanosis in severe cases

Complications
1. Secondary bacterial infection is very common
2. Bronchopneumonia
3. Cardiac failure, especially in the elderly

Treatment
1. Bed rest in a warm room with steam inhalations
2. Antibiotics such as tetracycline or penicillin
3. Codeine linctus to suppress troublesome cough

CHRONIC BRONCHITIS
Predisposing causes
1. Air pollution (i.e. urban environment)
2. Cigarette smoking
3. Dirty or dusty occupations
4. Obesity

Clinical features
1. 'Smoker's' cough with early morning sputum
2. Later a 'winter' cough develops, with wheezing and sputum which may be mucoid or purulent. These symptoms gradually become more persistent
3. Progressively increasing dyspnoea, with cyanosis

Complications
1. Cor pulmonale, with recurrent episodes of right ventricular failure
2. Bronchopneumonia

(contd.)

Respiratory system

Treatment
1. Avoidance of cigarette smoking, dusty work and obesity
2. Bronchodilators e.g. salbutamol
3. Antibiotics such as tetracycline or ampicillin should be given if the sputum becomes purulent
4. Sedative cough mixtures e.g. codeine linctus, will suppress cough at night. Expectorant cough mixtures may loosen sputum
5. Low concentration oxygen therapy for severe cases

EMPHYSEMA

A lung disease in which there is enlargement of the alveoli with destruction of their walls. Usually occurs in association with chronic bronchitis or chronic asthma. Patients are dyspnoeic on exertion, with a barrel-shaped chest which expands poorly

PNEUMONIAS

In pneumonia, alveolar inflammation causes the affected lung to become airless and solid with exudate (*consolidation*)

Organisms which commonly cause pneumonia
1. Streptococcus pneumoniae (pneumococcus)
2. Haemophilus influenzae
3. Mycobacterium tuberculosis (TB)
4. Staphylococcus aureus
5. Mycoplasma and viruses

LOBAR PNEUMONIA

This is localized to one or more lobes of the lungs. Pneumococcus is the commonest causative organism, and it often affects previously healthy adults

Clinical features of lobar pneumonia
1. Sudden onset of pyrexia and rigors or vomiting
2. Dyspnoea, with rapid shallow respiration and cyanosis
3. Cough with 'rusty' sputum
4. Pleuritic pain (worse on cough and deep breathing)
5. Herpes labialis (vesicles on lips)

Complications
1. Pleural effusion
2. Empyema
3. Cardiac failure
4. Septicaemia

BRONCHOPNEUMONIA

This has a more patchy distribution and spreads along the bronchioles. It is due to a variety of organisms (especially Haemophilus) and is often secondary to other disease. Young children and the elderly are most commonly affected

Predisposing causes
1. Bronchitis
2. Inhalation of infected material (e.g. mucus) or vomitus
3. Debilitation, with recumbency and poor respiratory movements
4. Pulmonary embolism or collapse

Clinical features

Resembles lobar pneumonia, but the onset is more gradual, cough and sputum are more variable, and pyrexia is irregular and resolves gradually

Complications
1. Cardiac failure
2. Pulmonary fibrosis

Treatment of bacterial pneumonia
1. Antibiotics according to bacterial sensitivity e.g. i.m. benzylpenicillin for pneumococcus
2. Pleuritic pain may require pethidine
3. Codeine will suppress irritant cough
4. High concentration oxygen therapy if central cyanosis develops

BRONCHIECTASIS

Dilatation of the bronchi, usually accompanied by recurrent bronchial suppuration

Causes
1. Complication of pulmonary collapse
2. Complication of pneumonia, especially TB or bronchopneumonia

Clinical features
1. Cough with profuse purulent sputum, especially on changing posture
2. Malaise, intermittent pyrexia, halitosis ('bad breath')
3. Weight loss (or 'failure to thrive' in a child)
4. Dyspnoea, often with cyanosis
5. Finger clubbing
6. Some patients have no symptoms

Complications
1. Recurrent pneumonia or pleurisy
2. Lung abscess or empyema
3. Septic emboli (p. 18)

Treatment
1. Frequent postural drainage
2. Antibiotics
3. Surgical removal of the affected lobe

INDUSTRIAL LUNG DISEASES

Pneumoconiosis is chronic lung disease due to inhalation of dusts by industrial workers

Types of pneumoconiosis
1. *Anthracosis,* in coal mines
2. *Silicosis,* in sand-blasters
3. *Siderosis,* in iron miners and foundry workers
4. *Asbestosis,* in workers with asbestos

Clinical features
Progressive dyspnoea, with cough and sputum

Complications
1. Pulmonary fibrosis
2. Emphysema
3. Cor pulmonale (cardiac failure secondary to lung disease)
4. Some types predispose to TB or cancer

ASTHMA

Intermittent bronchial spasm, often accompanied by sticky bronchial secretions. A severe attack lasting for many hours is called *status asthmaticus*

Predisposing causes
1. Many patients have an *atopic constitution* with a family history of asthma, infantile eczema, urticaria or hay fever. Such patients are often allergic to mites, pollens, animal hair, certain foods etc.
2. *Chronic bronchitis* and *respiratory tract infections*
3. *Psychological factors* e.g. stress at work, or tension in the home
4. Many cases develop in middle-age for no apparent cause (*idiopathic*)

Clinical features
1. Paroxysms of dyspnoea, with 'tightness' in the chest, and prolonged wheezy expirations
2. Cough (dry or with sticky plugs of sputum)
3. In severe cases, cyanosis and respiratory failure

Complications
1. Emphysema may develop in long-standing asthmatics
2. Recurrent chest infections

Treatment
1. *Antispasmodics* (drugs which relax the bronchial muscles)
   - i Aminophylline by i.v. injection or suppository
   - ii Isoprenaline ⎫
     Orciprenaline (*Alupent*) ⎬ by tablet or aerosol inhalers
     Salbutamol (*Ventolin*) ⎭

The excessive use of isoprenaline aerosols can cause death and patients must not exceed the recommended dose

2. *Corticosteroids*
ACTH, prednisone or hydrocortisone (p. 124) may be needed in severe cases. *Becotide Inhaler* delivers a potent glucocorticoid to the lungs with no danger of systemic side-effects

3. *Sodium cromoglycate (Intal)*
This may be administered regularly by a 'Spinhaler' to prevent asthma by inhibiting the release of bronchoconstrictor substances

4. *Antibiotics* e.g. tetracycline
These are used only if the sputum is infected

5. *Oxygen therapy* (p. 29)

OXYGEN THERAPY

This is used to correct tissue *hypoxia* (low oxygen tension)

Cyanosis is due to the presence of an excess of inadequately oxygenated haemoglobin in the blood

Peripheral cyanosis is limited to the extremities and is due to poor circulation (e.g. cardiac failure, or vasoconstriction due to cold)

Central cyanosis affects also the lips and tongue

Causes
1. Impaired oxygenation of blood in lungs
2. Congenital heart disease with a R. to L. 'shunt' of blood (e.g. Fallot's tetralogy)

High concentration oxygen therapy (40–80 per cent)

This is indicated in central cyanosis due to impaired gas exchange:
1. Shock e.g. myocardial infarction
2. Pulmonary oedema
3. Pneumonia
4. Cardiac failure

Suitable masks: Polymask or MC mask (Henley)

Low concentration oxygen therapy (25–40 per cent)

This is indicated in underventilation of the lungs due to chronic respiratory disease:
1. Chronic bronchitis
2. Emphysema
3. Severe, prolonged asthma

Suitable masks: Ventimask or Edinburgh mask

The administration of high conc. oxygen to a patient with carbon dioxide retention due to chronic respiratory disease may release the respiratory centre of the brain from its 'anoxic drive' and cause respiratory depression, with coma due to carbon dioxide narcosis. Only low conc. oxygen should be used in chronic respiratory disease

TUBERCULOSIS

In developed countries infection is with the human TB bacillus (*Mycobacterium tuberculosis*) which spreads by droplet infection in the atmosphere and affects the lungs

In under-developed countries infection with the bovine TB bacillus also occurs. This is transmitted in milk and causes abdominal TB

Primary TB is infection with the tubercle bacillus in a patient who has not previously been infected

Post-primary TB is re-infection or a recrudescence of the primary lesion

These 2 conditions follow different courses due to the increased immunological response in the post-primary disease

PRIMARY TB

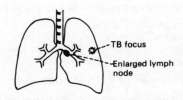

A small lesion occurs in any part of the lungs and the local hilar lymph nodes enlarge. The *Mantoux test* (intradermal injection of tuberculin) becomes positive. Most primary lesions heal spontaneously without complications, but occasionally pleural effusion or tuberculous bronchopneumonia may develop

POST-PRIMARY PULMONARY TB

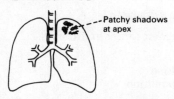
Patchy shadows at apex

The initial lesion is usually in the upper lobe of the lung but spread into other parts of the lung often follows. Necrosis of the affected part (*caseation*) may produce a cavity. The course is variable, depending on the patient's resistance. Healing may occur with fibrosis and calcification, but the disease usually slowly progresses unless halted by treatment

Clinical features
1. Early cases may have no symptoms
2. Malaise, pyrexia, anorexia, weight loss, tiredness or night sweats
3. Cough, may be dry or productive, sometimes with haemoptysis
4. In advanced cases, dyspnoea, cyanosis and wasting (cachexia)

Complications
1. Widespread tuberculous bronchopneumonia
2. Pleurisy, often with effusion or empyema
3. Massive haemoptysis
4. Blood-borne spread to another organ e.g. bone
5. Miliary TB (widespread dissemination throughout the body)

Treatment
1. Long-term chemotherapy with drugs such as streptomycin, isoniazid and sodium aminosalicylate (PAS), given in combination to prevent the emergence of resistant organisms
2. Adequate diet and rest
3. Surgical resection of affected lung in selected cases

Prevention
1. Improved hygiene and living conditions
2. Detection and isolation of patients with 'open' TB (i.e. bacilli in the sputum)
3. Vaccination with an attenuated strain of bacillus (BCG)

LUNG TUMOURS

1. BRONCHIAL CARCINOMA

This is the commonest cancer in Britain

Predisposing causes
1. Cigarette smoking
2. Atmospheric pollution

Clinical features
1. Cough, which may be dry or productive
2. Weight loss, malaise, anorexia
3. Chest pain, dyspnoea, haemoptysis

Common complications
1. Bronchial obstruction, with pulmonary collapse or infection (pneumonia or abscess)
2. Pleural effusion, often blood-stained
3. Obstruction of superior vena cava
4. Distant metastasis (spread to other organs)

Treatment
1. Surgical resection of the affected lung
2. Radiotherapy or cytotoxic drugs in selected cases

2. SECONDARY CARCINOMA

Cancer of other organs (e.g. breast) commonly spreads to the lungs (*pulmonary metastases*)

3. BRONCHIAL ADENOMA

An uncommon benign tumour which may cause haemoptysis or bronchial obstruction

PLEURISY

Inflammation of the pleura (the membrane which covers the lungs and lines the thoracic cavity) is called pleurisy

Pleurisy may be *dry* or associated with an *effusion* of fluid. The fluid may be serous (clear, straw-coloured), purulent or blood-stained. A collection of pus in the pleural cavity is called an *empyema*

Causes of pleural effusion
1. TB
2. Pneumonia or lung abscess
3. Bronchial cancer
4. Pulmonary infarct
5. Accompanying generalised fluid retention in severe cardiac, hepatic or renal failure

Clinical features

Dry pleurisy causes pain aggravated by cough and deep breathing
If *effusion* occurs the pain disappears but dyspnoea increases

PNEUMOTHORAX

Air in the pleural cavity

Causes
1. Traumatic
2. Iatrogenic e.g. during thoracic surgery
3. Spontaneous
   i In previous healthy young adults
   ii As a complication of emphysema or asthma

Clinical features
1. Pain in the chest, and dyspnoea
2. With a large pneumothorax the patient may be 'shocked'
3. The affected side is hyper-resonant to percussion, with diminished chest movement. The mediastinum may be pushed to the opposite side

Treatment
1. Patients who are shocked or in pain may need morphine
2. If the lung is collapsed a catheter is inserted into the pleural cavity, and connected to an under-water seal

BODY TEMPERATURE

The *temperature-regulating centre* is a group of neurones in the hypothalamus which act as a thermostat.

Normal oral temperature = 36.6 to 37.2°C (98 to 99°F)
Pyrexia = Above 37.2°C
Subnormal temperature = Below 36.6°C
Hypothermia = Below 35°C

The *rectal* temperature exceeds the *oral* temperature by 0.5°C
The *oral* temperature exceeds the *axillary* temperature by 0.5°C

Note that most thermometers take at least two minutes to register body temperature. If hypothermia is suspected (e.g. in a collapsed elderly patient) a special low-reading thermometer is required.

PYREXIA (FEVER)

Common causes

1. *Infection*
   Viral, bacterial or protozoal
2. *Malignancy*
   Carcinoma, leukaemia or lymphoma
3. *Hypersensitivity reaction*
   Hay-fever, drug reaction, 'collagen-vascular' disease (p. 114), etc.
4. *Infarction of tissue*
   Myocardial or pulmonary infarction

Spurious causes of pyrexia include taking a hot drink or a hot bath just prior to the temperature measurement.

Types of fever

Pyrexia may be *continuous* or *intermittent* (for only part of the day). A high intermittent fever suggests undrained suppuration, septicaemia or TB

A *rigor* is a bout of shivering seen in acute infections due to an increased setting of the hypothalamic 'thermostat'. It has three stages:

1. *Cold.* The patient shivers and feels cold, and the skin vessels are constricted
2. *Hot.* The patient is pyrexial, restless and thirsty, and may have a headache
3. *Sweating.* The patient sweats profusely and the symptoms subside as the temperature falls

Digestive system

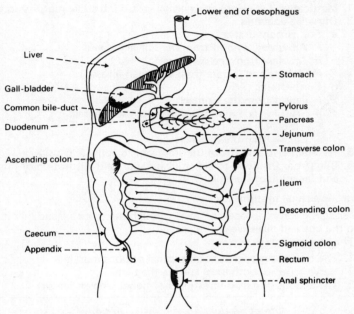

Gastro-intestinal tract from lower oesophagus to anus

In life the transverse colon lies just below the liver and in front of the pylorus

DIGESTION AND ABSORPTION

The function of the gastro-intestinal tract is to digest and absorb the following nutrients:
1. Carbohydrate, protein and fat
2. Vitamins
3. Minerals (especially sodium, calcium and iron)
4. Water

DIGESTION

Digestion (the breaking down of food into absorbable units) begins in the mouth and stomach and is completed in the small intestine

Requirements for digestion
1. Mastication (chewing) and normal gastro-intestinal motility (q.v.)
2. Digestive enzymes
   a For carbohydrates
      i Amylase (ptyalin) from the salivary glands
      ii Amylase from the pancreas
      iii Maltase and lactase from the small intestine
   b For proteins
      i Pepsin from the stomach
      ii Trypsin and chymotrypsin from the pancreas
   c For fats
      i Lipase from the pancreas
3. Hydrochloric acid (from the stomach) to activate pepsin
4. Bile (from the liver) to aid emulsification and absorption of fats and fat-soluble vitamins (D, A, K)

Gastro-intestinal motility

Peristaltic waves propel the food through the intestine and mix it with the bile and digestive enzymes
The mechanisms depend on:
1. The intrinsic properties of intestinal smooth muscle
2. Nerve reflexes, both local and via the brain
3. The actions of gastro-intestinal hormones (shown below)

Hormone	Site of production	Action
Gastrin	Pylorus and duodenum	Stimulates gastric acid secretion
Gastrozymin	Pylorus	Stimulates gastric enzyme secretion
Enterogastrone	Duodenum	Inhibits gastric secretion
Secretin	Duodenum	Stimulates watery secretion by the pancreas
Pancreozymin	Duodenum	Stimulates enzyme secretion by the pancreas
Cholecystokinin	Duodenum	Stimulates gall-bladder contraction

These hormones affect both digestive enzyme secretion and G.I. secretion and G.I. motility. Their actions overlap and interact in a complex way

ABSORPTION

The products of digestion are as follows:
1. Carbohydrates are broken down to three *monosaccharides* (glucose, galactose and fructose)
2. Proteins are broken down to *amino-acids*
3. Fats are broken down to *fatty acids and glycerol*

The absorptive surface of the small intestine is greatly increased by finger-like processes called *villi*. Each villus contains a network of *capillaries* and a blind-ended lymphatic (*lacteal*)

The capillaries absorb monosaccharides, amino-acids, minerals and water-soluble vitamins, and these are transported by the portal vein to the liver. The lacteals absorb digested fats and fat-soluble vitamins (D, A and K) and these are transported via the thoracic duct to the bloodstream

Water, sodium and chloride are absorbed in the colon

VITAMINS

Vitamins are complex chemicals, found in food in very small quantities, which are essential for health and development

Infants, pregnant women, alcoholics and elderly people living alone are particularly likely to develop a vitamin deficiency

Multiple vitamin deficiency with protein deprivation is common in developing countries, but it is unusual in the U.K. unless there is another factor such as alcoholism, malabsorption or a food fad

Vitamin A occurs in animal fats, eggs and carrots. Deficiency causes night blindness and dry painful eyes

Vitamin B complex occurs in eggs, peas, beans and cereals
1. *Thiamine* deficiency, which occurs where polished rice is the staple diet, causes *beri-beri* (heart failure and neuropathy)
2. *Riboflavine* deficiency causes *sore lips and tongue*
3. *Nicotinamide* deficiency occurs in the tropics and causes *pellagra* (diarrhoea, dementia and dermatitis)
4. *Cyanocobalamin* (B_{12}) deficiency causes *megaloblastic anaemia* and *subacute combined degeneration of the cord* (p. 97)

Vitamin C (ascorbic acid) occurs in fresh vegetables, especially citrus fruits, but it is destroyed by heat. Deficiency causes scurvy (anaemia, bleeding tendency, spongy gums and delayed healing)

Vitamin D (calciferol)
See p. 112

Vitamin K is found in green vegetables, and is also synthesized by bacteria in the intestine

Deficiency causes bleeding due to lack of clotting factors (prothrombin and factor 7)

THE MOUTH AND PHARYNX
The tongue
Pallor indicates anaemia

Dry brown tongue may occur in any severe illness, especially uraemia and acute intestinal obstruction

'Furring' may be due to smoking, or to many mild illnesses, especially gastro-intestinal upsets

Smooth, red tongue (atrophic glossitis) may be due to antibiotics, anaemia or vitamin deficiency

White patches may be due to Candidiasis (p. 108) or leukoplakia (thickened epithelium)

Causes of stomatitis (inflammation of the mouth)
1. Debilitation, excessive smoking, alcoholism
2. Infections
   - *i* Viral e.g. measles, herpes simplex
   - *ii* Bacterial e.g. pyorrhoea
   - *iii* Candidiasis ('thrush')
3. Iron or vitamin deficiency

Mouth toilet is especially important in denture-wearers and in dehydrated patients

Causes of dysphagia (difficulty in swallowing)
1. Painful conditions of mouth or pharynx e.g. stomatitis, tonsillitis
2. Paralysis of muscles of pharynx e.g. poliomyelitis
3. Foreign body in the oesophagus or pharynx
4. Disease of the oesophagus e.g. cancer
5. Compression of oesophagus e.g. by thyroid or bronchial cancer

THE STOMACH
Functions of the stomach
1. Storage of food after a meal
2. Mixing of food with gastric secretions
3. Controlled release of the resulting mixture (chyme) into the duodenum
4. Secretion of pepsin
5. Secretion of hydrochloric acid
6. Secretion of intrinsic factor, an enzyme necessary for B_{12} absorption in the terminal ileum

Digestive system 39

Common causes of anorexia (loss of appetite)
1. Malignancy
2. Gastro-intestinal disorders e.g. gastritis
3. Cardiac, hepatic or renal failure
4. Drugs e.g. digoxin
5. Depression or anxiety
6. Chronic illness, especially if painful

Causes of vomiting
1. *Feeding upsets:* (in babies) and *dietary indiscretions*
2. *Intra-abdominal disease*
    - *i* Inflammation
      e.g. Gastric ulcer
           Gastro-enteritis
           Peritonitis
           Pancreatitis
           Cholecystitis
           Hepatitis
    - *ii* Obstruction (p. 44)
3. *Cerebral*
    - *i* Motion sickness
    - *ii* Migraine
    - *iii* Labyrinthitis
    - *iv* Raised intra-cranial pressure
4. *Psychological* e.g. disgust, fear, pain
5. *Metabolic*
    - *i* Pregnancy
    - *ii* Febrile illness e.g. tonsillitis (especially in children)
    - *iii* Uncontrolled diabetes

Types of vomitus
1. Food, usually partly digested
2. Fluid, which may be bile-stained (greeny-black)
3. Blood (haematemesis)—bright red if recent
   dark brown ('coffee-grounds') if old
4. Faeculent—dark brown, foul-smelling fluid due to prolonged intestinal obstruction

Projectile vomiting, in which the gastric contents are ejected with great force, occurs in pyloric stenosis

Causes of haematemesis
1. Peptic ulcer or gastritis
2. Aspirin ingestion
3. Oesophageal varices (dilated veins due to portal hypertension)
4. Hiatus hernia

HIATUS HERNIA

A portion of the upper end of the stomach protrudes through the oesophageal opening of the diaphragm into the thorax

Clinical features
1. Dyspepsia (indigestion), especially on lying down
2. Bleeding may cause haematemesis or anaemia

Treatment
1. Weight reduction
2. Small meals and antacids
3. Sleeping in 'head-up' position
4. In severe cases, surgical repair of the diaphragm

DYSPEPSIA

Causes
1. Defective teeth, hurried or irregular meals
2. Dietary indiscretion (excess alcohol, pickles, etc.)
3. Organic disease
    i Hiatus hernia
    ii Gastritis or gastric carcinoma
    iii Peptic ulcer
    iv Disease of liver or gall-bladder
    v Heart failure

Clinical features
1. Flatulence (epigastric discomfort, distension and belching)
2. Heart-burn (pain behind the sternum)
3. Water-brash (regurgitation of fluid into the mouth)
4. Nausea and vomiting

PEPTIC ULCER

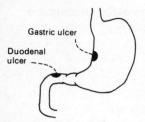

The common sites for peptic ulcer

GASTRIC ULCER

Clinical features
1. Epigastric pain, usually localized, and occurring soon after food
2. Vomiting, which often relieves the pain
3. Epigastric tenderness

DUODENAL ULCER

Clinical features resemble gastric ulcer but:
1. The pain may wake the patient in the night and is relieved by food
2. Vomiting is less common in duodenal ulcer
3. Duodenal ulcer is more common in men

Complications of peptic ulcers
1. Bleeding.
   Massive haematemesis may cause collapse
   Small bleeds may cause anaemia
2. Perforation
3. Obstruction due to scarring ('hour glass stomach')

Medical treatment of peptic ulcers
1. Adequate rest and removal of anxiety
2. Stop smoking and avoid aspirins
3. Antacids e.g. magnesium trisilicate or aluminium hydroxide
4. Anticholinergic drugs (to diminish gastric peristalsis) e.g. propantheline
5. Carbenoxelone ('Biogastrone' for gastric ulcer, 'Duogastrone' for duodenal ulcer) speeds healing
6. Dietary modification where necessary

FAECES

These normally consist of unabsorbed food residue, bacteria and water

1. **Quantity**

    Copious stools occur in malabsorption
    Scanty stools occur in dehydration

2. **Colour**

    The normal brown colour is due to bile pigments

    Pale stools are due to
      i   Biliary tract obstruction
      ii Excessive fat (malabsorption)
    Dark grey stools occur after iron ingestion
    Black tarry stools (melaena) are due to bleeding in the upper gastro-intestinal tract
    Red blood in the stools is seen in bleeding from the colon or rectum (e.g. ulcerative colitis, cancer of colon or haemorrhoids)
    Pus in the stools occurs in colitis, dysentery and burst pelvic abscess

3. **Consistency**

    Liquid stools occur in diarrhoea
    Hard lumpy stools occur in constipation
    Slimy stools (due to mucus) occur in diseases of the colon
    Foreign bodies or *parasites* such as roundworms, threadworms and tapeworms may also be noted

4. **Odour**

    Very malodorous stools occur in malabsorption

Some characteristic abnormal stools:

1. *Malabsorption*
    Soft, pale, bulky stools, often oily, malodorous and difficult to flush away
2. *Dysentery*
    Watery stools mixed with red blood and pus
3. *Cholera*
    Pale watery stools, free of odour, with shreds of epithelium and mucus ('Rice-water')
4. *Intussusception*
    'Red-currant jelly'

DIARRHOEA
Frequent passage of unformed motions
Causes
Acute
1. Dietary indiscretion e.g. excessive beer
2. Food poisoning e.g. toadstools, Staphylococcal toxins
3. Gastro-intestinal infection
    i Viral 'gastro-enteritis'
    ii Bacterial e.g. typhoid fever or bacillary dysentery
    iii Protozoal e.g. amoebic dysentery
4. Psychogenic e.g. nervousness
5. Drugs e.g. purgatives and antibiotics

Chronic
1. Intestinal inflammation
    i Ulcerative colitis
    ii Diverticulitis
    iii Carcinoma of colon
2. Malabsorption (q.v.)
3. Metabolic e.g. thyrotoxicosis

'Spurious' diarrhoea can follow the impaction of solid faeces in the elderly

MALABSORPTION
Causes
1. Gastrectomy or removal of part of the ileum
2. Biliary tract obstruction
3. Pancreatic failure (chronic pancreatitis or fibrocystic disease)
4. Coeliac disease (flat jejunal mucosa due to gluten allergy)
5. 'Blind-loop' syndrome after intestinal surgery, (due to overgrowth of bacteria in the gut)

ABDOMINAL COLIC
'Griping' abdominal pain due to spasmodic contraction of the intestine
Causes
1. Indigestible foods e.g. unripe apples
2. Gastro-enteritis
3. 'Irritable bowel' syndrome ('functional')
4. Intestinal obstruction
5. Purgatives and poisons

CONSTIPATION

Delay in evacuation of faeces.
Many patients are unduly worried about constipation. Many normal people defaecate only once in three days, others as often as three times daily

Causes
Acute
1. Paralytic ileus
    i Abdominal surgery
    ii Peritonitis
    iii Acute febrile illness (e.g. pneumonia)
2. Obstruction (q.v.)

Chronic
1. Ineffective peristalsis
    i Dehydration or lack of solid food
    ii Chronic purgation
    iii Metabolic e.g. hypothyroidism
    iv Drugs e.g. codeine
2. Obstruction (q.v.)
3. Dyschezia (distended insensitive rectum due to persistent failure to respond to the desire to defaecate)

INTESTINAL OBSTRUCTION

Common causes
1. Adhesions from previous operation
2. Strangulated hernia
3. Volvulus (twisted intestine)
4. Intussusception (invagination of the intestine)

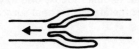

5. Tumour e.g. carcinoma of colon

ASCITES

Fluid accumulation in the peritoneal cavity

Causes
1. Peritoneal inflammation
    i Secondary cancer deposits
    ii TB
2. Increased pressure in portal vein
    i Cirrhosis
    ii Congestive heart failure
    iii Constrictive pericarditis
3. Generalized oedema e.g. nephrotic syndrome

ACUTE GASTRO-ENTERITIS
Causes
1. Ingestion of bacterial toxins e.g. Staphylococcal
2. Ingestion of poisons e.g. toadstools
3. Allergy to a particular food
4. Bacterial infection e.g. Salmonella typhi-murium
5. Viral infection

Clinical features
1. Malaise
2. Nausea and vomiting
3. Abdominal colic
4. Diarrhoea

Infantile gastro-enteritis may cause severe toxaemia and dehydration necessitating i.v. fluids

REGIONAL ILEITIS (CROHN'S DISEASE)
Patchy inflammation, often starting in the terminal ileum, with thickening of the intestinal wall and narrowing of the lumen. The cause is unknown

Clinical features
1. Usually young adults
2. Malaise, weakness, weight loss, pyrexia
3. Intermittent abdominal pain with tenderness in R. iliac fossa
4. Mild or moderate diarrhoea

Complications
1. Obstruction
2. Perforation
3. Abscess
4. Fistula

Treatment
1. Broad spectrum antibiotics
2. Prednisone
3. Surgical resection of the affected bowel

ULCERATIVE COLITIS

The mucosa of the colon becomes thick, inflamed and ulcerated. The cause is unknown, but some patients have an obsessional personality

Clinical features

1. Often in middle adult life (3rd or 4th decade)
2. Malaise, weakness, weight loss, pyrexia
3. Diarrhoea with blood and mucus. Often severe and chronic
4. Pain in L. iliac fossa

Complications

1. Perforation
2. Haemorrhage, dehydration, loss of electrolytes
3. May develop cancer of colon in later life

Treatment

1. Bed rest with a high-calorie, high-protein diet supplemented by vitamins and oral iron
2. Sulphasalazine (*'Salazopyrine'*) or prednisone orally
3. Correction of severe anaemia or electrolyte loss by transfusion or i.v. fluids
4. Surgery for severe cases (ileostomy or colectomy)

DIVERTICULITIS

Multiple blind sacs (diverticula) form in the wall of the sigmoid colon. This is called *diverticulosis* if the sacs are asymptomatic, but *diverticulitis* if they become inflamed

Clinical features

1. Usually middle-aged or elderly
2. Recurrent bouts of colicky abdominal pain
3. May be either constipation or diarrhoea
4. Tenderness in L. iliac fossa, often with a palpable mass

Complications

1. Obstruction
2. Perforation
3. Abscess
4. Fistula into bladder or vagina

Treatment

1. Analgesics
2. Broad-spectrum antibiotics e.g. tetracycline
3. Surgery for severe cases e.g. colostomy

THE LIVER

Structure

The liver consists of an enormous number of lobules, each about 1 mm in diameter.

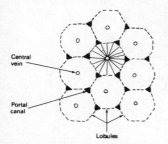

Each portal canal contains branches of the hepatic artery, the portal vein and a bile ductule

Each lobule consists of a mass of cubical liver cells arranged in columns as shown below, but the lobules are not clearly demarcated.

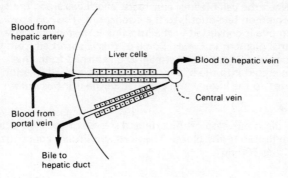

Functions of the liver

1. Formation of bile pigments (from Hb) and bile salts
2. Carbohydrate metabolism—formation and storage of glycogen
3. Fat metabolism
4. Formation of plasma proteins, especially albumin and clotting factors
5. Urea formation by breakdown of proteins
6. Storage of vitamins A and B_{12}
7. Inactivation of some hormones, drugs and toxins

Entero-hepatic circulation

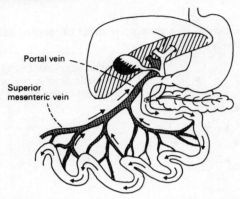

Bile is secreted into the biliary canaliculi in the liver. It leaves the liver by the hepatic ducts and is stored and concentrated in the gall-bladder. When the gall-bladder contracts, bile flows along the cystic duct and common bile-duct into the duodenum. The *conjugated bilirubin* in bile is converted in the intestine into *stercobilinogen* which is the normal pigment in faeces. Some of this is absorbed from the intestine into the portal blood stream and returned to the liver. Most of this is re-excreted into the bile by the liver, but a small fraction escapes and is carried to the kidney and excreted in the urine as *urobilinogen*

JAUNDICE

Yellow discolouration of the skin and sclerae of the eyes due to increased bilirubin in the blood. The normal bilirubin concentration is less than 1 mg/100 ml

Causes
1. Obstruction of biliary tract (cholestasis)
   i In the lumen—gall stones
   ii In the wall—cholangitis
   iii Pressure from outside—cancer in liver, lymph nodes, pancreas, stomach
2. Hepatic cellular failure
   i Hepatitis
   ii Cirrhosis
   iii Toxins e.g. carbon tetrachloride (used in dry-cleaning)
3. Haemolysis

VIRAL HEPATITIS
Cause
Two strains of virus cause an identical clinical picture
1. Virus A—transmitted in stools
   Incubation period 3—6 weeks
2. Virus B (Serum hepatitis)—transmitted by blood (transfusion, accidental inoculation etc.) which contains the Australia antigen
   Incubation period 3—6 months

Clinical features
1. Fever, malaise, anorexia
2. Jaundice develops a few days later
3. Large tender liver
4. Intra-hepatic biliary obstruction (due to cellular oedema) causes pale stools with dark urine
5. Depression and tiredness often persist after recovery

Treatment
Bed-rest with a low-fat diet and avoidance of alcohol

CIRRHOSIS
Fibrosis and nodular regeneration of the liver with impaired hepatic function

Causes
1. Many cases are idiopathic
2. Alcoholism
3. Following viral hepatitis

Clinical features
1. Due to hepatic failure
   - *i* Jaundice and 'spider naevi' (dilated arterioles with tiny vessels radiating from them)
   - *ii* Bleeding tendency (due to deficiency of prothrombin)
   - *iii* Tremor, lethargy and confusion (hepatic encephalopathy)
   - *iv* Weight loss and dyspepsia
   - *v* Oedema
2. Due to portal hypertension:
   - *i* Bleeding from dilated oesophageal veins (varices)
   - *ii* Ascites

Treatment
1. Avoidance of alcohol
2. For oedema, a low-salt diet with spironolactone
3. Surgery (porta-caval shunt) may be considered for the relief of portal hypertension

CHOLECYSTITIS

Inflammation of the gall-bladder, may be acute or chronic

Clinical features
1. Usually obese middle-aged patients
2. Nausea, vomiting, flatulence, fever
3. Epigastric pain, especially after fatty foods
4. Tenderness over gall-bladder, especially on deep inspiration

Treatment
1. Analgesics
2. Broad-spectrum antibiotics e.g. tetracycline

CHOLELITHIASIS

Gall-stones, often form in chronic cholecystitis

Clinical features
1. May be asymptomatic
2. Biliary colic (excruciating epigastric pain, often with vomiting)
3. Obstructive jaundice

THE PANCREAS
FUNCTIONS
Exocrine secretions
1. *Digestive enzymes*
   i Trypsinogen and chymotrypsinogen
   ii Amylase
   iii Lipase
2. *Sodium bicarbonate.* This neutralizes the acid secretions from the stomach

Endocrine secretions
1. *Glucagon* from the α cells (p. 90)
2. *Insulin* from the β cells (p. 90)

ACUTE PANCREATITIS
Cause
Unknown, but may follow pancreatic duct obstruction or excess of alcohol

Clinical features
1. Severe upper abdominal pain
2. Vomiting and 'shock'

Treatment
1. Analgesics e.g. pethidine
2. Intravenous fluids as necessary for 'shock'

CHRONIC PANCREATITIS
Follows recurrent acute pancreatitis

Clinical features
1. Malabsorption (weight loss and pale fatty stools)
2. Diabetes mellitus

Treatment
1. Low-fat diet and avoidance of alcohol
2. *Pancreatin* (enzymes) orally with meals

Nervous system

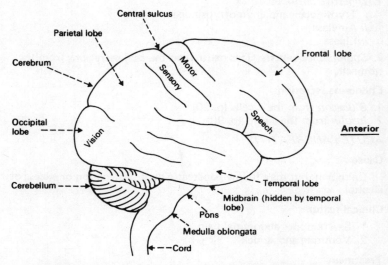

The *cerebrum* has psychic, motor and sensory functions. The two cerebral hemispheres each send and receive impulses from the opposite side of the body

Movements are initiated by the *motor cortex,* anterior to the central sulcus

Sensations are received by the *sensory cortex,* posterior to the central sulcus

Vision is transmitted by the optic nerves and optic tract to the occipital lobe

The *speech centre* is located in Broca's area in the frontal lobe of the dominant hemisphere (in a R. handed person this is the L. hemisphere)

The *cerebellum* maintains posture and regulates muscular tone and activity

The *midbrain, pons and medulla* contain nerve tracts connecting cerebrum, cerebellum and spinal cord, and they contain important centres such as the respiratory and vasomotor centres and most of the cranial nerve nuclei

CRANIAL NERVES

- 1st, *Olfactory,* conveys smell sensation
- 2nd, *Optic,* conveys vision from retina to brain
- 3rd, *Oculomotor* ⎫
- 4th, *Trochlear* ⎬ regulate eye-movement
- 6th, *Abducens* ⎭
- 5th, *Trigeminal,* conveys sensation from face and scalp
- 7th, *Facial,* supplies facial muscles and conveys taste
- 8th, *Auditory,* conveys sensation of hearing and balance
- 9th, *Glossopharyngeal* ⎫ supply pharynx and larynx to regulate
- 10th, *Vagus* ⎬ swallowing and voice production
- 11th, *Spinal Accessory,* supplies some neck muscles
- 12th, *Hypoglossal,* supplies the muscles of the tongue

Common cranial nerve lesions
Optic neuritis

Degeneration or inflammation of the 2nd Cr. N. may cause misty vision and painful eye movements

Ophthalmoplegia

Paralysis of ocular movement due to lesions of 3rd, 4th or 6th Cr. Ns. May be accompanied by:
1. *Strabismus* (squint)
2. *Diplopia* (double vision)
3. *Ptosis* (drooping eyelid)

Trigeminal neuralgia

Paroxysmal attacks of excruciating pain in the distribution of the 5th Cr. N.

Facial palsy

7th Cr. N. paralysis

Causes
1. 'Stroke' affecting internal capsule (often with hemiplegia)
2. Bell's palsy (of unknown cause)
3. Trauma to facial nerve, or pressure on nerve e.g. from parotid tumour

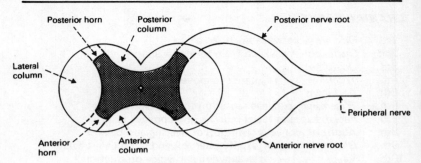

Transverse section of spinal cord

MOTOR PATHWAY

Fibres from neurones (*upper motor neurones*) in the motor cortex cross over in the medulla and descend in the lateral column of the spinal cord. These fibres end in the anterior horn and relay (synapse) with the anterior horn cells (*lower motor neurones*) which transmit impulses to the muscles via the anterior nerve root and peripheral nerve

SENSORY PATHWAY

Sensory impulses from the peripheral nerve endings enter the spinal cord by the posterior horn. Fibres conveying position, vibration and touch travel upwards in the posterior column of the cord and cross over at the medulla. Fibres carrying pain and temperature cross over at once and travel upwards in the anterior and lateral columns. All these sensory fibres relay in the thalamus, whence impulses are conveyed to the sensory cortex

REFLEX ACTION

Reflex action allows rapid responses e.g. withdrawal from heat. A sensory stimulus passes into the posterior horn of the spinal cord and is conveyed directly to the motor cells of the anterior horn so that a movement is made without any conscious effort by the subject. Tendon reflexes such as the knee jerks are used to test the function of the nervous system

ABNORMALITIES OF MOVEMENT

A. *LOSS OF MOVEMENT*

Paralysis is the inability to move a particular muscle
Paresis is weakness of a muscle short of complete paralysis
Monoplegia is paralysis of one limb
Hemiplegia is paralysis of the arm and leg on one side of the body
Paraplegia is paralysis of both legs

Causes of paraplegia
1. Congenital defect of brain ('spastics')
2. Trauma to spinal cord (vertebral fracture, etc.)
3. Compression of the spinal cord
   i Neoplasm of cord or meninges
   ii Abscess
   iii Vertebral disease (TB, osteoma, etc.)
4. Degenerative disease of the cord
   i Disseminated sclerosis
   ii 'Sub-acute combined degeneration' due to vit. B_{12} deficiency

Spasticity and flaccidity

Lesions of the *upper motor neurones* in the brain (p. 54) or their descending fibres in the spinal cord cause *spastic paralysis,* with rigid limbs and exaggerated tendon reflexes

Lesions of the *lower motor neurones* in the anterior horn (p. 54) or their fibres in the peripheral nerves cause *flaccid paralysis* with limp limbs and absent tendon reflexes

B. *INVOLUNTARY MOVEMENT*

1. **Tremor** (shaking)

   Causes
   i Parkinsonism
   ii Cerebellar disease
   iii Alcoholism
   iv Thyrotoxicosis

2. **Spasm** (involuntary contraction of a muscle)

   Causes
   i Epilepsy
   ii Disseminated sclerosis
   iii Tetanus

   In *tonic spasm* the muscle remains contracted
   In *clonic spasm* the contractions are rhythmical

3. **Choreiform movements**

   Short jerky movements seen in chorea (p. 10)

4. **Athetosis**

   Refers to slow writhing movements, usually caused by brain damage

C INCOORDINATION OF MOVEMENT

This is called *ataxia*

Causes
1. Alcoholic intoxication
2. Cerebellar disease
3. Tabes dorsalis (syphilis)

THE CEREBROSPINAL FLUID

The c.s.f. which bathes the brain and spinal cord is secreted by the choroid plexuses into the ventricles of the brain. It then passes through three small openings in the roof of the brain stem (behind the pons) into the *subarachnoid space* (p. 57)

Changes in c.s.f. may help in diagnosis:
1. Turbid or purulent c.s.f. occurs in *meningitis*. The organism may be identified by culture
2. Blood in c.s.f. occurs in *subarachnoid haemorrhage*
3. C.s.f. pressure is increased by *cerebral tumour* and *haematoma*
4. Proteins in c.s.f. may be increased in *cerebral tumour* and *disseminated sclerosis*
5. The c.s.f. Wassermann reaction is positive in *syphilis*

HYDROCEPHALUS

Failure of communication between the ventricles of the brain and the subarachnoid space results in accumulation of c.s.f. with consequent dilatation of the ventricles. In infants the brain is flattened, the skull enlarges and mental deficiency may ensue

Causes
1. Congenital defect
2. Meningitis

THE MENINGES

The three membranes which surround the brain and spinal cord:
1. *Dura mater* (outer layer)
2. *Arachnoid*
3. *Pia mater* (inner layer)

The c.s.f. occupies the sub-arachnoid space (between the arachnoid and pia mater)

MENINGITIS

Inflammation of the meninges

Causes
1. Bacterial
    i Meningococcal
    ii Tuberculous
    iii Pyogenic e.g. Pneumococcus, Streptococcus, Haemophilus

2. Viral

Clinical features common to all types of meningitis
1. Fever, malaise and vomiting
2. Headache, neck stiffness and backache
3. Drowsiness, delirium, coma

Specific features

Meningococcal—a severe form, often accompanied by a purpuric rash. Some cases develop septicaemia, with bleeding into the adrenal glands, and consequent 'shock'

Tuberculous—often of more gradual onset and running a longer course. Many cases have permanent after-effects

Pyogenic—may be an extension of infection from the middle ear or nasal sinuses

Viral—tends to be relatively mild

Complications of meningitis
1. Cranial nerve palsy
2. Focal cerebral lesions e.g. paralysis
3. Epilepsy
4. Hydrocephalus

POLIOMYELITIS

A viral infection which destroys motor neurones in the anterior horn of the cord and the cranial nerve nuclei (p. 53). It is transmitted by droplet infection and in the faeces, but is becoming rare in U.K. due to vaccination

Clinical features
1. Usually children or young adults
2. Sudden onset of an influenza-like illness, often with headache and stiff neck
3. After a few days either these symptoms subside or paralysis rapidly develops. Recovery is gradual, but permanent weakness is common and the affected muscles become atrophic
4. The brain stem may be affected with paralysis of swallowing and respiration ('bulbar polio')

Treatment
1. Strict barrier nursing and bed rest, preferably in a 'polio unit'
2. Physiotherapy, with splints and supports, is required if paralysis develops. Analgesics and sedatives may be needed
3. In bulbar polio the patient may need tracheostomy, suction, positive-pressure ventilation etc.

NEUROSYPHILIS

About 10 per cent of patients with syphilis develop neurological disease some years after the primary infection.

There are three main types:

1. Meningo-vascular syphilis

Inflammation of the vessels to the meninges and brain causes a wide variety of CNS lesions with headache, confusion, epilepsy, localising signs etc.

2. Tabes dorsalis

Degeneration of the fibres in the posterior columns of the spinal cord may cause sharp stabbing leg pains, unsteady gait, impotence, optic atrophy, deep skin ulcers and destructive, painless arthritis (Charcot's joints)

The pupils are small, irregular and do not constrict when tested with light (Argyll Robertson pupils)

3. General paralysis of the insane (G.P.I.)

Insidious onset of dementia (intellectual deterioration) and personality change, usually in middle-aged men. Dysarthria, tremors and spastic weakness are common

The diagnosis of these three diseases is usually confirmed by finding a positive Wasserman Reaction (W.R.) and characteristic protein changes in the cerebro-spinal fluid

Treatment of neurosyphilis

Intramuscular penicillin, repeated until the W.R. becomes negative

COMA
Loss of consciousness
Causes
1. Head injury
2. Epilepsy
3. Drugs e.g. alcohol, anaesthetic, hypnotics
4. Syncope (q.v.)
5. Cerebro-vascular accident (p. 62)
6. Cerebral tumour
7. CNS infection e.g. meningitis, abscess
8. Severe metabolic disturbance
   - *i* Hypoglycaemia
   - *ii* Diabetic ketosis
   - *iii* Uraemia
   - *iv* Hepatic failure

Syncope is a transient loss of consciousness due to inadequate cerebral blood-flow
Causes
1. Vaso-vagal attack ('faint')
2. Massive bleeding
3. Stokes-Adams attack (heart-block)

INTRA-CRANIAL TUMOUR
The terms *'intra-cranial tumour'* and *'space-occupying lesion'* are often used synonymously to include all expanding lesions inside the skull

Causes
1. Neoplasm
2. Abscess
3. Haematoma

Common intra-cranial neoplasms
1. Glioma (malignant, arising from cerebrum)
2. Meningioma (benign, arising from meninges)
3. Secondary metastases (malignant, often from breast or bronchus)

Clinical features of intra-cranial neoplasm
1. Localizing effects, depending on the site. May be motor, sensory or psychic
2. Raised intra-cranial pressure
   - *i* Headache (worse on straining) and drowsiness
   - *ii* Bradycardia
   - *iii* Vomiting
   - *iv* Papilloedema (swelling and blurring of the optic disc)
3. Epilepsy

EPILEPSY

A paroxysmal disturbance of brain function which ceases spontaneously and tends to recur

Predisposing causes
1. Birth injury and cerebral malformation
2. Cerebral tumour
3. Trauma
4. Cerebro-vascular accident
5. Infection e.g. encephalitis or meningitis
6. Metabolic upset
    - *i* Exhaustion and stress
    - *ii* Anoxia
    - *iii* Hypoglycaemia
    - *iv* Pyrexia, especially in children

    Many cases are idiopathic

Symptoms of epilepsy
1. Loss of consciousness (partial or complete)
2. Convulsive movements
3. Sensory abnormalities
4. Autonomic disturbance, especially incontinence
5. Psychic disturbance

Types of epilepsy

1. Grand mal

The classical epileptic fit has the following stages:
- *i* *Aura*—the patient is aware a convulsion is imminent
- *ii* *Tonic*—sudden coma with generalized rigidity and absent respiration
- *iii* *Clonic*—convulsive movements, salivation and incontinence
- *iv* *Coma*—the limbs are limp with absent reflexes
- *v* *Recovery of consciousness*—may be accompanied by headache, or automatism in which the patient is unaware of his actions

2. Petit mal

A brief interruption of consciousness in which the patient may only stop what he is doing for a few seconds

3. Focal epilepsy

Clinical features depend on the site affected. In temporal lobe epilepsy there may be bizarre movements, emotions or sensations

4. Status epilepticus

A series of grand mal seizures without intervening recovery of consciousness. May be fatal if untreated

Treatment of epilepsy

Treatment of a 'grand mal' attack
1. Place a gag between the teeth to prevent tongue biting
2. Loosen the collar and maintain the airway
3. Restrain only to prevent self-injury   (contd.)

Prophylactic treatment

Drugs must be taken regularly to reduce the frequency of attacks

    e.g. Phenobarbitone } for grand mal
         Phenytoin

       Ethosuximide, for petit mal

Treatment of 'status epilepticus'

Diazepam (Valium) by slow i.v. injection, or paraldehyde by i.m. injection.

CEREBRO-VASCULAR DISEASE

A *'stroke'* (cerebro-vascular accident) may be due to:

1. **Intra-cranial haemorrhage**
2. **Cerebral ischaemia** due to thrombosis, embolism or spasm of the carotid, vertebral or cerebral vessels. The embolus commonly arises from a damaged heart (e.g. mitral stenosis or myocardial infarct)

'Strokes' may be of slow or sudden onset, and of all degrees of severity from slight transient weakness to sudden death. They commonly affect the internal capsule of the brain and cause hemiplegia or hemiparesis of the opposite side of the body, often with dysphasia

Dysphasia refers to difficulty in the use of words, whether spoken or heard. Dysphasic patients recognize objects, but cannot think of the name for them

Dysarthria refers to difficulty in the articulation of words.

Dysarthric patients cannot speak clearly, e.g. due to painful tongue, cerebellar lesions etc.

Sites of intra-cranial haemorrhage
1. **Extra-dural haemorrhage**

Usually a ruptured meningeal artery due to a skull fracture. Produces rapidly progressing coma due to cerebral compression. Immediate operation to relieve the pressure is required

2. **Sub-dural haematoma**

Usually follows a minor head injury in elderly patients, with blood oozing from veins into the sub-dural space. After a latent period of some days there is gradual onset of headaches, drowsiness, weakness and eventual coma

3. **Subarachnoid haemorrhage**

Usually a ruptured cerebral aneurysm (dilated artery). Severe headache, often occipital, followed by coma

4. **Intracerebral haemorrhage**

Clinical features vary depending on the site and size of the bleed

MIGRAINE

The attacks are due to transient constriction, followed by dilatation, of the branches of the external carotid artery

Clinical features
1. An 'aura' precedes the attack e.g. flashing lights, numbness or tingling
2. Paroxysmal headache, usually confined to one side of the head
3. Attacks are often accompanied by vomiting and photophobia (dislike of the light)

Factors which may precipitate migraine
1. Emotional upset or anxiety
2. Overwork
3. Certain foods e.g. chocolate
4. Fluid retention e.g. due to oral contraceptives, or premenstrually

Treatment
1. Avoidance of precipitating causes. *Sedation* or *Clonidine* may help to prevent attacks
2. *Ergotamine tartrate* should be given early in each attack, either dissolved under the tongue or as a suppository or intramuscular injection

PARKINSONISM

The pathological lesion is degeneration of the *basal ganglia* of the brain. There is also depletion of a neurotransmitter called *dopamine*

Causes
1. Idiopathic 'paralysis agitans'
2. Drugs, especially phenothiazines (e.g. chlorpromazine) in high dosage
3. As a late sequel of encephalitis

Clinical features
1. Insidious onset in elderly patients
2. Immobile face
3. Shuffling gait with characteristic posture
4. Tremor, which is most marked at rest
5. Rigidity (resistance to passive movement of a joint)

Treatment

Useful drugs include:
1. *Laevodopa,* which is converted into dopamine in the brain
2. *Amantadine* (*Symmetrel*)
3. *Benzhexol* (*Artane*)

DISSEMINATED SCLEROSIS

The pathological lesion is patchy demyelination (loss of white matter) of the central nervous system but the cause is unknown

Clinical features
1. Onset is in young adults, insidious but gradually progressive over many years
2. Spastic weakness, usually starting in legs
3. Sensory loss or paraesthesiae (tingling)
4. Diplopia (double vision) or optic neuritis (p. 53)
5. Cerebellar signs
    i Slow staccato speech
    ii Intention tremor e.g. on picking up a pin
    iii Nystagmus (oscillating eye movements)
6. Eventually mental changes, paraplegia with painful spasms and sphincter changes occur

Treatment
ACTH or cyanocobalamin injections may help

MOTOR NEURONE DISEASE

An uncommon disease of unknown cause in which progressive degeneration of the anterior horn cells in the spinal cord and the upper motor neurones in the brain causes muscle wasting and weakness

SYRINGOMYELIA

An uncommon disease of unknown cause in which cavities develop in the spinal cord, causing progressive weakness, wasting and loss of pain and temperature sensation

DISORDERS OF PERIPHERAL NERVOUS SYSTEM
NEURITIS
This term refers to all types of peripheral nerve disease (degenerative, traumatic or inflammatory). The term neuropathy is more accurate

Causes
1. Many cases are idiopathic
2. Bacterial infection e.g. leprosy, tetanus
3. Trauma e.g. compression by crutches or stretching
4. Vitamin deficiency, especially B_{12}
5. Miscellaneous metabolic upsets
    - *i* Diabetes mellitus
    - *ii* Chronic uraemia
    - *iii* Bronchial carcinoma

Clinical features
1. Weakness or paralysis
2. Numbness or tingling, often in a 'glove and stocking' distribution
3. Trophic changes e.g. muscle wasting or skin ulcers
4. Loss of tendon reflexes
   The localization depends on which nerves are affected

Polyneuritis affects many nerves symmetrically and simultaneously. If progressive and severe this can be fatal due to paralysis of respiratory muscles

Carpal tunnel syndrome

Pain and tingling in the fingers due to compression of the median nerve at the wrist

Causes of muscle wasting
1. Part of cachexia (generalized wasting) in severe illness such as cancer or TB
2. Atrophy due to disease of a muscle e.g. in arthritis or limb-splinting
3. Disease of the anterior horn cells or peripheral nerves e.g. polio, motor neurone disease, peripheral neuropathy

MYASTHENIA GRAVIS

A rare disease in which a defect of synthesis and storage of acetylcholine at the nerve-muscle junction causes muscles to tire very rapidly. Treatment with *neostigmine* restores the power by preventing the breakdown of acetylcholine at motor nerve-endings. Thymectomy may help

MUSCULAR DYSTROPHY

A group of uncommon inherited diseases in which muscles degenerate with consequent loss of power. Sometimes the muscles become bulky (pseudohypertrophy) despite their weakness

INSOMNIA

Inability to sleep

COMMON CAUSES

1. Physical factors
    - *i* Pain or discomfort
    - *ii* Dyspnoea
    - *iii* Cough
    - *iv* Frequency of micturition
    - *v* Flatulence
    - *vi* Pruritus
    - *vii* Restlessness associated with a febrile illness
    - *viii* Withdrawal of hypnotic drugs
2. Psychological factors
    - *i* Worry or anxiety
    - *ii* Excitement (may be induced by drugs or coffee)
    - *iii* Depression (especially early morning waking)
    - *iv* Psychiatric illness e.g. hallucinations
3. Environmental factors
    - *i* Noise
    - *ii* Light
    - *iii* Hard bed
    - *iv* Cold or excess heat

Urinary system

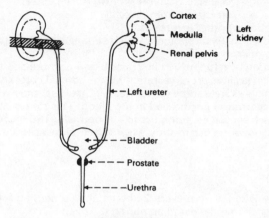

Male renal tract

Each kidney contains about one million functional units called *nephrons* (shown below). The *glomeruli* receive blood at high pressure from the afferent arterioles and the fluid filtered from the blood (*glomerular filtrate*) passes down the *tubules* to the *renal pelvis.* During its passage, the tubules selectively reabsorb various constituents (water, sodium, potassium, glucose, etc.) of the glomerular filtrate to maintain the composition of the body fluids constant.

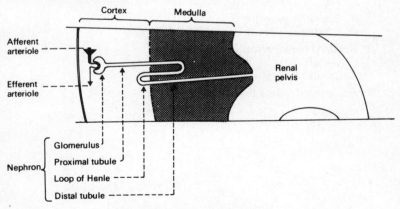

Arrangement of a nephron
(Diagrammatic view of the area shaded above in the right kidney)

FUNCTIONS OF THE KIDNEY
1. Maintenance of tissue fluids at constant composition
2. Excretion of end-products of metabolism—
    e.g. urea from protein breakdown
           uric acid from breakdown of cell nuclei
           creatinine from muscle
3. Excretion of drugs and toxins
4. Secretion of erythropoietin, which stimulates red cell production in the marrow
5. Secretion of renin, which increases blood pressure and also stimulates aldosterone secretion by the adrenal cortex (p. 89)

The kidneys excrete some substances (e.g. glucose) only when a certain concentration is exceeded in the blood. This *threshold value* varies for each substance. For glucose it is normally 180 mg/100 ml of blood, and glycosuria occurs only when this level is exceeded

URINE

QUANTITY

Normally ½ to 2½ litres every 24 hours, the production rate being much greater during the day than during the night

Causes of polyuria (increased urine production)
1. Excessive fluid intake (especially alcohol or coffee)
2. Chronic renal failure
3. Diabetes mellitus or diabetes insipidus
4. Diuretic drugs

Causes of oliguria (decreased urine production)
1. *Dehydration*
    i Decreased fluid intake
    ii Excessive sweating
    iii Diarrhoea, vomiting, gastric aspiration
2. *Reduced renal perfusion*
    i 'Shock'
    ii Cardiac failure
3. *Acute renal failure* (p. 74)

COLOUR

Varies, depending on concentration and on the amount of urochrome pigment. Fresh urine should be clear, but it may 'cloud' on standing. Cloudiness of fresh urine may be due to pus, bacteria or phosphates

Causes of dark urine

1. *Blood*

    Small quantities give a smoky appearance
    Large quantities give a reddish-brown colour

2. *Bile or excessive urobilin*
3. *Ingested dyes*
    - i Natural e.g. rhubarb, beetroot
    - ii Synthetic e.g. coloured sweets, phenolphthalein
4. *Rare metabolic diseases* e.g. porphyria

SPECIFIC GRAVITY

The normal urine S.G. is 1.001 to 1.025 at room temperature
The specimen passed on rising should exceed 1.020
In renal failure the urine S.G. is constant at 1.010
Substances which increase the urine S.G.—
   1. Urea or chloride
   2. Glucose
   3. Albumin

REACTION

The pH of normal urine is neutral or slightly acid

CHEMICAL TESTING OF URINE

1. **Protein**

    The urine should be clear before testing, so it may need filtering
    Albustix: Dip strip in urine and remove immediately

Yellow	=	negative
Green—blue	=	positive

2. **Blood**

    Occultest: 1 drop of urine on test paper + 1 tablet + 2 drops of water will produce a blue colour if blood is present

    Haematuria (red cells in urine) is distinguished from *haemoglobinuria* (Hb without red cells) by microscopy

(contd.)

3. Sugars

The most important is glucose (glycosuria);
Clinistix: Dip strip in urine
Blue = positive
This test is sensitive and specific for glucose but it gives no idea of quantity

Clinitest: 5 drops of urine + 10 drops of water + 1 tablet in test-tube. Watch until boiling stops, then shake gently and compare with colour chart.

Light-green	=	0.1 to 0.5%
Green	=	0.5 to 1%
Yellow	=	1 to 2%
Red	=	over 2%

This test is quantitative, but it detects glucose, lactose and fructose

4. Bile

Bile causes a yellow froth on shaking the specimen
Ictotest: 5 drops of urine on test mat + 1 tablet + 2 drops of water
Bluish-purple colour around the tablet = positive

5. Urobilin

This is formed in the intestine during the enterohepatic circulation of bile (p. 48)

Absence of urobilin from urine indicates complete biliary tract obstruction

Excess of urobilin is due to:
  i Haemolysis (with excess bilirubin from Hb breakdown)
  ii Hepatic failure (inability of the liver to re-excrete urobilin)
Test by adding *Ehrlich's aldehyde reagent* and heating:
  Normal urine turns red
  Absence of red colour on heating = absence of urobilin
  Presence of red colour before heating = excessive urobilin

6. Ketones

The ketones (acetone and two more complex molecules) are derived from the excessive breakdown of fats. If they occur in the urine the patient is said to be ketotic.
Acetest: 1 drop of urine + 1 tablet
Mauve = positive

Causes of proteinuria

1. *Contamination*
   In women, with *vaginal secretion*
   In men, with *semen* or *prostatic secretion*
2. *'Postural'* (orthostatic) proteinuria
   Disappears when the patient is horizontal, and is absent from the specimen passed on rising. It does not indicate disease
3. *Renal disease*
   i Glomerulonephritis, especially in nephrotic syndrome
   ii Pyelonephritis
   iii Malignant hypertension
   iv Tuberculosis
4. *Disease of renal tract* e.g. cystitis
5. Slight albuminuria often occurs in *fevers* or in *congestive heart failure*
6. Patients with *multiple myeloma* secrete Bence-Jones protein, which coagulates on heating but redissolves on boiling

Causes of haematuria

1. *Kidney lesions*
   i Trauma
   ii Glomerulonephritis, pyelonephritis or TB
   iii Hypernephroma
2. *Renal tract lesions*
   i Cystitis or bladder tumour
   ii Calculi from kidney or bladder
   iii Prostatic disease, especially carcinoma
3. *Bleeding disease or anticoagulant overdose*

Causes of glycosuria

1. Hyperglycaemia (glucose over 180 mg/100 ml blood)
2. Low renal threshold (defective tubular reabsorption)

Causes of ketosis

1. Starvation
2. Uncontrolled diabetes mellitus
3. Prolonged vomiting

Urine microscopy

This may reveal—
1. Red cells
2. Pus cells (leucocytes)
3. 'Casts' of the renal tubules
4. Bacteria
5. Parasites (e.g. Schistosoma)

MICTURITION

The emptying of the bladder is normally controlled by the nervous system. A full bladder (300—400 ml) stimulates impulses along the afferent fibres to the sacral part of the spinal cord. The micturition reflex is normally inhibited by the brain until a convenient time, when efferent impulses from the spinal cord contract the bladder musculature and simultaneously the urethral sphincter muscle relaxes

DISORDERS OF MICTURITION

A. Incontinence (absence of voluntary control)

Causes

1. Infancy
2. Nocturnal enuresis (bed-wetting during sleep)
3. Coma or epileptic fit
4. Spinal cord injury or disease (e.g. tumour)
5. 'Stress incontinence', due to weakness of the pelvic floor muscles or urethral sphincter. Any rise of intra-abdominal pressure (e.g. laughing, coughing, sneezing) causes a leak of urine

B. Retention of urine

Common causes in the male

1. Post-operative
2. Prostatic enlargement
3. Urethral stricture

Common causes in the female

1. Trauma of labour
2. Pressure on bladder neck from uterus enlarged by pregnancy or a fibroid

Other causes in both sexes include:

i Stones (from kidney or bladder)
ii Neoplasm of bladder
iii Clot (bleeding from kidney or bladder)
iv Spinal cord injury or disease (e.g. disseminated sclerosis)

It is most important to distinguish *urine retention* from *anuria* (p. 74) **'Retention with overflow'**. As the bladder becomes hugely distended the pressure forces open the sphincter and small quantities of urine leak out periodically. The distended bladder is easily felt as a firm round mass above the pubis

Urinary system 73

C. Frequency of micturition

Causes

1. *Polyuria* (p. 68)
2. *'Irritation'* of the bladder or urethra
   - *i* Cystitis
   - *ii* Calculus
   - *iii* Pressure from pregnancy or pelvic tumour
3. *Anxiety* (e.g. before interview or examination)

D. Dysuria (painful micturition)

Causes

1. Pyelonephritis
2. Cystitis
3. Urethritis

E. Hesitancy, poor stream and dribbling

In *hesitancy* the urine flow is delayed after voluntary relaxation of the sphincter

A *poor stream,* due to partial urethral obstruction, prolongs micturition

Dribbling implies continuing leakage of drops of urine after the end of micturition

These three symptoms are characteristic of prostatic hypertrophy

RENAL FAILURE

This may be acute or chronic

In *acute* failure the kidneys may produce little urine (*oliguria*) or no urine (*anuria*)

In *chronic* failure they may fail to respond to antidiuretic hormone (p. 85) leading to the constant production of large quantities of dilute urine of fixed specific gravity (usually 1.010)

Metabolic effects of renal failure

1. *Uraemia* (blood urea exceeding 40 mg/100 ml) due to accumulation of protein metabolites
2. *Hyperkalaemia* due to potassium retention
3. *Hyponatraemia* due to loss of sodium in urine
4. *Hypoproteinaemia* due to loss of albumin in urine
5. *Hypocalcaemia* due to loss of calcium in urine
6. *Acidosis* (decreased blood pH)

'URAEMIA'

This term is often used to refer to the overall clinical picture of advanced renal failure

Clinical features of 'uraemia'

1. Loss of energy, drowsiness, confusion
2. Anorexia, nausea, vomiting, hiccups
3. Pruritus, pallor and 'earthy' pigmentation
4. 'Air hunger' (Kussmaul breathing) due to acidosis (p. 21)
5. Cardiac arrhythmia or cardiac arrest, due to hyperkalaemia
6. Osteomalacia or secondary hyperparathyroidism, due to hypocalcaemia

ACUTE RENAL FAILURE

Causes

1. 'Shock'
    i Blood loss or fluid loss
    ii Hypotension e.g. myocardial infarction
    iii Septicaemia
    iv Obstetric disasters e.g. abortion or ante-partum haemorrhage
2. Acute glomerulonephritis or pyelonephritis
3. Severe crush injuries

Clinical features

1. Oliguria (urine output below 500 ml/24 hours)
2. 'Uraemia' (see above)

(contd.)

Urinary system

Treatment
1. Correction of fluid and electrolyte loss. For an adult the fluid intake is about 500 ml plus the volume of urine passed in the previous 24 hours. It is usually given as a concentrated glucose solution to supply calories to minimize tissue breakdown
2. An anabolic steroid to minimize tissue breakdown
3. Resonium A (binds potassium in the intestine) to lower plasma potassium
4. If necessary, peritoneal dialysis or haemodialysis

If recovery of renal function occurs the patient enters a *diuretic phase,* with large volumes of dilute urine. Large amounts of water, sodium and potassium are lost and may need to be replaced

GLOMERULONEPHRITIS

This term is applied to diffuse inflammatory disease affecting the glomeruli. It is probably due to complex immunological reactions to a variety of antigenic stimuli, including infection with β-haemolytic streptococci or viruses. It is classified by the histological appearance of a renal biopsy specimen:
1. **Minimal change**—changes seen only on electron microscopy
2. **Membranous**—diffuse thickening of the glomerular capillary walls
3. **Proliferative**—increased number of cells in all glomeruli
4. **Focal**—proliferative changes seen in only some parts of some glomeruli

There are two main clinical types of glomerulonephritis:
1. *Acute nephritis*
2. *Nephrotic syndrome*

Either can develop hypertension or progress to chronic renal failure, and many intermediate types occur

ACUTE NEPHRITIS

Clinical features
1. Often youngsters with a history of Streptococcal tonsillitis one to three weeks previously
2. Sudden onset of headache, pyrexia, vomiting, loin pain
3. Scanty urine, with albuminuria and a smoky appearance due to haematuria
4. Moderate oedema, often periorbital, and worse in the morning

Prognosis

Most cases recover completely in a few weeks, but some die of acute renal failure or develop progressive chronic renal failure

Treatment
1. Bed rest
2. Penicillin for a few days to eradicate Streptococci
3. High calorie diet, with restriction of protein, fluid and salt until the diuretic phase occurs

NEPHROTIC SYNDROME

This is characterized by:
1. Heavy proteinuria
2. Low plasma proteins
3. Massive oedema

Glomerulonephritis is by far the commonest cause of the nephrotic syndrome but it is occasionally secondary to other disease e.g. diabetes

Clinical features
1. Insidious onset of oedema, with a pale puffy face. The oedema becomes generalized, often with ascites or pleural effusion
2. Increased susceptibility to infections

Prognosis

Variable, but oedema may persist for months or years. Many patients ultimately develop renal failure

Treatment
1. High protein diet with restriction of salt
2. Diuretics (p. 119)
3. Prednisone or immunosuppressive drugs such as azathioprine
4. Paracentesis (drainage) of ascites or pleural effusion

CHRONIC RENAL FAILURE

Common causes
1. Glomerulonephritis
2. Pyelonephritis
3. Malignant hypertension
4. Urinary tract obstruction e.g. stones or prostatic enlargement

Clinical features
1. *Nocturia* (increased nocturnal urine production) is an early symptom, followed eventually by *polyuria*
2. 'Uraemia' develops insidiously (p. 74)

Treatment
1. Fluid intake should be at least 3 litres daily, because in chronic renal failure the excretion of urea etc., is proportional to the urinary flow. Salt supplements may be needed
2. Low protein diet (e.g. 40 g daily). In more advanced cases the Giovanetti diet is used, with vitamin supplements
3. Blood transfusion may be needed for severe anaemia
4. Hypertension should be controlled (p. 7)
5. Dialysis with artificial kidney or renal transplant should be considered

URINARY TRACT INFECTION

The urinary tract consists of the renal pelvis, ureter, bladder and urethra.

CYSTITIS

Inflammation of the bladder, usually due to bacterial infection

Common bacterial causes
1. *Escherischia coli*
2. *Streptococcus faecalis*
3. *Proteus vulgaris*
4. *Pseudomonas pyocyaneus*

It predominantly affects women, since the short female urethra readily allows bacteria to spread from the perineum to the bladder

Infection can also descend from an infected kidney, and conversely infection of the lower urinary tract is often followed by acute pyelonephritis

Other predisposing causes:
 i Retention of urine
 ii Calculi
 iii Bladder diverticula or cancer

Clinical features
1. Frequency of micturition, with dysuria
2. Cloudy urine with offensive odour
3. May be rigors, pyrexia and supra-pubic tenderness

ACUTE PYELONEPHRITIS

Infection of the renal pelvis, often also involving the kidney tissue

Predisposing causes
1. Lower urinary tract infection, especially if accompanied by urinary stasis (e.g. pregnancy, prostatic hypertrophy, paraplegia etc.)
2. Reflux of urine up the ureters due to urethral or ureteric dysfunction
3. Pre-existing renal disease
4. Pre-existing systemic disease e.g. diabetes mellitus

Clinical features
1. Sudden onset of fever, rigors and malaise
2. Pain and tenderness in one or both loins
3. Frequency, dysuria and cloudy offensive urine

Treatment of cystitis and acute pyelonephritis
1. High fluid intake
2. Antibacterial drugs according to bacterial sensitivity e.g. sulphonamides, cotrimoxazole, ampicillin, nalidixic acid or nitrofurantoin (p. 123)
3. Sodium bicarbonate to keep the urine alkaline

Follow-up urine cultures are essential to ensure the infection is eradicated. The underlying cause should be treated if possible since recurrent infection can lead to fatal chronic pyelonephritis

CHRONIC PYELONEPHRITIS

The pathogenesis is poorly understood but recurrent infection seems to produce small scarred kidneys and eventual renal failure. In some cases the onset is insidious with sterile urine and no history of urinary tract infection

Clinical features
1. May resemble acute pyelonephritis
2. Asymptomatic proteinuria for years, followed by progressive renal failure

Treatment
1. Prolonged treatment (several months) with appropriate antibacterial drugs according to sensitivity
2. Treatment of renal failure (p. 76)

Renal failure is often precipitated by an exacerbation of the infection or an electrolyte disturbance (e.g. from prolonged vomiting)

CALCULI

Calculi (stones) may form either in the kidney or the bladder, and they usually consist of calcium salts, phosphates, urates or mixtures Factors which predispose to stone formation:
1. Excess calcium in the urine e.g. hyperparathyroidism
2. Excess urates in the urine e.g. gout
3. Urinary tract infections e.g. cystitis
4. Stasis of urine e.g. prostatic enlargement

Clinical features
1. A stone may produce no symptoms if it remains in the kidney
2. A stone entering the ureter produces *renal colic* (paroxysmal severe pain in the loin radiating into the abdomen and groin), often with haematuria. The patient is often restless, sweating and vomiting
3. A stone in the bladder may cause dysuria and frequency
4. Small stones may pass uneventfully through the urethra. Larger ones may lodge and cause retention of urine

Treatment
1. For renal colic, morphine or pethidine may be needed
2. Stones may pass naturally but failing this, operative removal may be required
3. Correction of predisposing cause

Reproduction

FEMALE REPRODUCTIVE SYSTEM

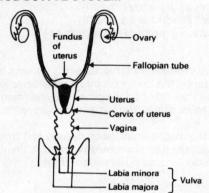

Diagram of female genitalia

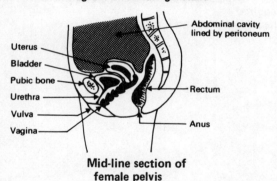

Mid-line section of female pelvis

The menstrual cycle, ovulation and conception

Menstruation, which starts at puberty, is controlled by the cyclical release of *gonadotrophins* (LH and FSH) from the anterior pituitary (p. 85). The menstrual flow lasts 3 to 5 days, and recurs at regular intervals of about 28 days until the menopause at age 40 to 50.

(contd.)

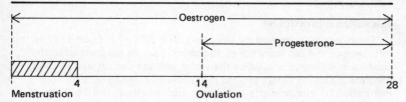

The menstrual cycle

The ovaries produce oestrogen throughout the cycle. Every month in midcycle (day 14) one of the two ovaries produces an ovum from a *follicle*. The follicle matures during the first half of the cycle under the influence of FSH and on day 14 the mature ovum is expelled and enters the fallopian tube (oviduct). The follicle is then converted into a *corpus luteum* which secretes progesterone to prevent further ovulation. If the ovum is fertilized by a sperm it embeds itself in the uterine wall and the corpus luteum continues to produce progesterone. No menstruation occurs and the symptoms of early pregnancy (morning sickness, breast tingling etc.) develop. If the ovum is not fertilized, however, the corpus luteum degenerates and shedding of the endometrium (uterine lining) starts on day 28.

A short rise in body temperature occurs shortly after ovulation. Timing intercourse to coincide with this rise may, therefore, help a woman to become pregnant.

MALE REPRODUCTIVE SYSTEM

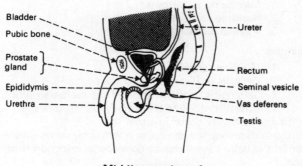

Mid-line section of male pelvis

Spermatazoa production

Testosterone is formed by the interstitial cells of the testis under the influence of the pituitary gonadotrophins. Sperms are formed in the coiled *seminiferous tubules* of the testis, and are then stored in their millions in the vas deferens until ejaculation of *semen* occurs.
Formation of sperms starts at puberty and continues until old age. If sexual intercourse or masturbation does not occur, spontaneous discharge of semen may occur in the sleep ('wet dream').

Sex of the fetus

During the formation of sperms and ova a 'reduction division' occurs so that the chromosomes are halved. Females have XX chromosomes so each ovum carries only one X. Males have XY chromosomes so each sperm carries either X or Y. The resulting fetus is, therefore, either XX or XY depending on the chromosome carried by the successful sperm.

VENEREAL DISEASES

Diseases transmitted by sexual intercourse

GONORRHOEA

Infection by the gonococcus (*Neisseria gonorrhoea*)
Incubation period 3 to 10 days

Clinical features

Male:
1. Purulent urethral discharge
2. Scalding on micturition
3. Tender lymph nodes in the groin

Female:
1. May be no symptoms
2. Scalding on micturition
3. Vaginal discharge

Complications

Male:
1. Urethral stricture
2. Orchitis (inflammation of the testis)

Female:
1. Salpingitis (inflammation of the Fallopian tubes)
2. Infertility (due to blocked Fallopian tubes)

Arthritis and rash may occur in either sex

Gonorrhoea in pregnancy can cause *ophthalmia neonatorum* (infection of the baby's eyes) due to gonococcal infection from the birth canal

Treatment of gonorrhoea

A single large dose of i.m. penicillin will cure most cases, but resistant gonococci may need another antibiotic such as kanamycin

SYPHILIS

Infection by a spirochaete (*Treponema pallidum*)
Incubation period 3 to 5 weeks

Clinical features of acquired syphilis

In the adult there are three stages:

1. *Primary syphilis*
The site of infection (e.g. penis, vulva, cervix, rectum, nipple or mouth) develops a hard painless 1 cm ulcer called a *chancre,* and the regional lymph nodes enlarge

2. *Secondary syphilis*
This develops about 6 weeks later, and can persist for up to 2 years:
   - *i* Tiredness, malaise, fever, sore throat, headache
   - *ii* Slight generalized lymphadenopathy
   - *iii* A non-irritable maculo-papular rash, often involving palms and soles
   - *iv* Condylomata lata (moist warty papules) around the genitalia or anus
   - *v* Patchy alopecia

3. *Tertiary syphilis*
This develops 2 to 20 years from the onset, after a latent period free from symptoms. It may take several forms:
   - *i* Cardiovascular syphilis, e.g. aortitis
     aortic incompetence
     aortic aneurysm
   - *ii* *Neurosyphilis* (p. 59)
   - *iii* *Gumma* (granulomatous inflammation) of skin, bone, liver or testis

Congenital syphilis

Infection of the baby via the placenta is now rare in the U.K. due to routine *Wasserman Reaction* (W.R.) blood tests in ante-natal clinics. Congenital syphilis can cause abortion, still-birth, deafness, blindness, rash, deformed bones and teeth, etc.

Diagnosis of syphilis

In primary syphilis the spirochaete can be found in the chancre. In secondary and tertiary syphilis the W.R. is positive

Treatment

Penicillin injections for 10 days. The course may need to be repeated until the W.R. becomes negative

TRICHOMONAS VAGINALIS

This is a protozoon which causes *vaginal discharge* in women and *balanitis* (inflammation of the foreskin) in men. Treatment is with metronidazole (Flagyl) orally, which should also be given to the sexual partner

NON-SPECIFIC URETHRITIS

The cause is unknown, but it may be due to a virus or mycoplasma

Clinical features
1. Frequency and scalding on micturition
2. Urethral discharge

Complications

Some patients develop *Reiter's syndrome,* with arthritis, conjunctivitis and a rash

Treatment

Tetracyclines may help

Endocrinology

Exocrine glands produce an external secretion via a duct e.g. sweat, sebaceous, lacrimal and mammary glands

Endocrine glands secrete hormones ('chemical messengers') into the blood

THE PITUITARY GLAND

The pituitary lies in the pituitary fossa, just above and behind the nasal cavity. The *hypothalamus* regulates pituitary activity by a series of *'releasing'* and *'inhibiting'* factors which pass along small blood vessels (the portal tract) linking the hypothalamus to the pituitary. The pituitary hormones control most of the other endocrine glands, and their hormones, in turn, have a *'negative feed-back'* effect on the hypothalamus

The **anterior** pituitary secretes the following hormones:
1. *Thyrotrophin* (TSH) stimulates the thyroid
2. *Corticotrophin* (ACTH) stimulates the adrenal cortex
3. *Somatotrophin* (Human growth hormone, HGH) stimulates growth
4. *Melanocyte stimulating hormone* (MSH) stimulates pigmentation
5. *Gonadotrophins* stimulate the gonads
    - i Follicle-stimulating hormone (FSH) in the female, and interstitial cell-stimulating hormone (ICSH) in the male
    - ii Luteinizing hormone (LH)
6. *Somatomammotrophin* (prolactin, luteotrophin) stimulates the mammary glands

The **posterior** pituitary secretes the following hormones:
1. *Antidiuretic hormone* (ADH) stimulates water reabsorption by the renal tubules
2. *Oxytocin* initiates labour and enhances uterine contractions

HYPERPITUITARISM

Pituitary over-activity, usually due to a pituitary adenoma (benign tumour)

Excessive HGH during childhood causes *gigantism* with an eventual height of 7 or 8 feet

Excessive HGH during adult life causes *acromegaly* with large hands and feet, characteristic coarse features, jutting jaw and thick greasy skin

The pressure of a pituitary adenoma on the optic chiasma (crossing of the optic nerves) may cause loss of vision

HYPOPITUITARISM
Pituitary under-activity

Causes
1. Pituitary necrosis following severe haemorrhage during pregnancy or childbirth
2. Non-secreting adenoma
3. Pituitary destruction by surgery or irradiation

Clinical features

In *children*, dwarfism and failure of sexual maturation
In *adults*:
1. Loss of body hair, loss of libido and cessation of menstruation
2. Pale thin skin
3. Hypothyroidism (p. 87)
4. Hypoadrenalism (p. 90)

Diabetes insipidus

Lack of ADH secretion by the posterior pituitary leads to the production of large volumes of dilute urine and frequent thirst

THE THYROID GLAND

The thyroid, which consists of two lobes connected by an isthmus, secretes two hormones:

1. *Thyroxine* stimulates tissue metabolism. It increases oxygen consumption and heat production
   Over-production of thyroxine causes hyperthyroidism
   Under-production of thyroxine causes hypothyroidism
   A person producing the normal amount of thyroxine is said to be *euthyroid*
2. *Calcitonin* increases calcium deposition in bone, but its importance is uncertain

GOITRE

A thyroid enlargement which may or may not secrete excess thyroxine

A 'toxic' goitre is overactive and causes thyrotoxicosis

With a 'non-toxic' goitre the patient remains euthyroid, but the goitre may press on the trachea or oesophagus

Causes of a 'non-toxic' goitre
1. A temporary goitre is common at puberty and during pregnancy
2. Iodine deficiency
3. Many cases are idiopathic

HYPERTHYROIDISM (THYROTOXICOSIS)

Clinical features
1. Goitre which may be diffuse or nodular
2. Fine tremor
3. Warm moist skin and intolerance of heat
4. Weight loss, increased appetite and diarrhoea
5. Rapid bounding pulse
6. Tiredness and nervousness
7. May be exophthalmos (protruding eyeballs)

Treatment
1. Antithyroid drugs e.g. thiouracil, carbimazole
2. Partial thyroidectomy, especially for large goitres
3. Radio-iodine is used in older patients

HYPOTHYROIDISM (MYXOEDEMA)

Causes

Primary (Thyroid gland failure)
1. Autoimmune thyroiditis
2. Iatrogenic:
    i Surgery
    ii Irradiation
    iii Excessive antithyroid medication
3. Cretinism (dwarfism and mental deficiency due to congenital hypothyroidism) is due to maternal iodine deficiency

Secondary
TSH deficiency due to pituitary failure

Clinical features
1. Mental and physical sluggishness
2. Dry rough skin with sparse hair and periorbital puffiness
3. Croaking voice and slow speech
4. Cold intolerance
5. Weight gain, constipation
6. Bradycardia (slow pulse)

Treatment

Maintenance with 0.3 mg l-thyroxine daily. A much lower dose may be advisable initially to avoid precipitating cardiac failure

THE PARATHYROIDS

The pea-sized glands, embedded in the posterior aspect of the thyroid, which secrete *parathormone*

Action of parathormone on calcium metabolism

There is an inverse relationship between the levels of calcium and phosphate in the blood, so that as phosphate falls, calcium increases

Parathormone acts on the renal tubules to increase the loss of phosphate in the urine. This lowers the phosphate level in the blood and to compensate for this the blood calcium is increased by increasing calcium mobilization from the bones. The net result of parathormone is to increase the serum calcium at the expense of the bones

HYPERPARATHYROIDISM

Parathormone excess

Causes
1. Parathyroid adenoma or hyperplasia (overactivity)
2. Parathyroid overactivity secondary to chronic renal failure or osteomalacia

Clinical features
1. Anorexia, constipation and thirst due to hypercalcaemia (increased blood calcium)
2. Renal stone due to increased urinary calcium and phosphate excretion
3. Bone pain, deformity and fractures due to thinning of bones

Treatment

Surgical: partial parathyroidectomy or removal of the adenoma

HYPOPARATHYROIDISM

Parathormone deficiency

Usually follows accidental removal of the parathyroids during thyroidectomy. The resulting hypocalcaemia causes *tetany*

Clinical features
1. Paraesthesiae ('pins and needles') of digits
2. Muscle spasm of hands and feet. The spasm is increased by applying a tourniquet to the limb (Trousseau's sign)
3. Increased tendon reflexes
4. May be convulsions, especially in children

Tetany may also result from *acidosis* due to the depletion of carbon dioxide in the blood by over-breathing

Treatment

Tetany due to hypocalcaemia is abolished by the slow intravenous injection of calcium gluconate

Thereafter, dietary supplements of calcium and vitamin D

THE ADRENAL GLANDS

These two glands lie immediately above the kidneys. Each gland has 2 parts:
1. The central *medulla* secretes the catecholamines, *noradrenaline* and *adrenaline*
2. The outer *cortex* secretes a variety of *steroid* hormones

Noradrenaline is the chemical transmitter at sympathetic nerve endings
It thus causes vasoconstriction and raises the blood pressure

Adrenaline prepares the body for physical activity—the 'fight, fright or flight' reaction. Its actions include:
1. Dilatation of pupils and bronchioles
2. Constriction of sphincters and inhibition of peristalsis
3. Acceleration of heart rate and increase in cardiac contractile force
4. Breakdown of liver glycogen with a consequent rise in blood glucose

Steroid hormones

1. *Mineralocorticoids*

Aldosterone conserves body sodium by stimulating sodium re-absorption in the renal tubules. The blood volume is probably regulated by the complicated *renin-angiotensin* system as follows—

A fall in blood volume produces a fall in blood pressure. This stimulates the kidneys to secrete renin which converts a circulating plasma protein called angiotensinogen into angiotensin. Angiotensin stimulates the release of aldosterone from the adrenals, which produces sodium retention, and this results in an increase in the osmotic pressure of the tissue fluids. This releases ADH from the posterior pituitary and the diminution in urine flow results in water retention and an increased blood volume.

2. *Glucocorticoids*

Cortisol (hydrocortisone) has several effects
   i It is anti-inflammatory and anti-allergic
   ii It increases protein breakdown and decreases the use of carbohydrates
   iii It increases sodium and water retention

Cortisol is secreted at times of stress, e.g. during infections or after an injury, as a result of ACTH release from the pituitary

3. *Sex hormones*

Small amounts of *testosterone*, *oestrogen* and *progesterone* are synthesized by the adrenal cortex

CUSHING'S DISEASE

Overactivity of the adrenal cortex

Causes
1. Hyperplasia secondary to pituitary overactivity
2. Adenoma or rarely adrenal carcinoma

Clinical features
1. Obesity of trunk and face, often with plethoric complexion and hirsutism
2. Hypertension
3. Striae (stretch-marks), easy bruising and pigmentation
4. Muscle weakness and bone thinning, often with vertebral collapse

Treatment

Surgical. Usually adrenalectomy but some cases secondary to pituitary disease require hypophysectomy

Adrenal tumours which secrete excess sex hormones can cause precocious puberty in children or virilization in women

HYPOADRENALISM

Underactivity of the adrenal cortex

Causes
1. Addison's disease (auto-immune adrenalitis)
2. Adrenal tuberculosis
3. Prolonged glucocorticoid therapy (e.g. prednisone) causes 'adrenal suppression'

Clinical features
1. Debility and tiredness
2. Nausea and vomiting
3. Pigmentation affecting palmar areas and mouth
4. Low blood pressure

Treatment

Daily hormone replacement with cortisone, with fludrocortisone to increase sodium retention

THE PANCREAS

In addition to its exocrine secretions (p. 51), the pancreas produces two hormones

1. *Glucagon,* produced by the α-cells, increases blood glucose by increasing the breakdown of liver glycogen
2. *Insulin,* produced by the β-cells, decreases blood glucose by inhibiting glycogen breakdown and facilitating the entry of glucose into tissue cells

DIABETES MELLITUS

A metabolic disorder in which the tissues fail to use glucose, which results in *hyperglycaemia* (increased blood sugar) and *glycosuria* (excretion of sugar in the urine)

Since the tissues cannot use glucose to provide energy, fats are broken down at an increased rate and this causes *ketosis* (excessive formation of ketones, p. 70)

Causes
1. Usually idiopathic. Predisposing factors include obesity and a family history of diabetes. In young patients an auto-immune mechanism may operate, and these cases of 'juvenile diabetes' are often very severe
2. Occasionally secondary to:
    - *i* Other disease e.g. pancreatitis, acromegaly
    - *ii* Drugs e.g. prednisone, diuretics

Clinical features
1. Weight loss and weakness due to inability to use glucose
2. Polyuria (increased urine production) due to the osmotic effect of glucose in urine
3. Thirst due to the polyuria

Complications
1. *Ocular*
    - *i* Cataract (opacity in the lens)
    - *ii* Retinopathy (haemorrhage, exudate, retinal detachment, etc.)
2. *Neurological*
   Numbness and paraesthesiae, especially in the lower limbs
3. *Renal*
   Pyelonephritis and glomerulonephritis
4. *Vascular*
   Occlusion of vessels may cause gangrene of feet, myocardial infarction or 'stroke'
5. *Infections*
   Increased susceptibility to:
    - *i* Boils and carbuncles
    - *ii* Candidiasis ('thrush'), which may cause vulval itching
    - *iii* Tuberculosis
6. *Coma*
    - *i* Diabetic ketosis (q.v.)
    - *ii* Hypoglycaemia (q.v.)

DIABETIC KETOSIS

This condition is characterized by hyperglycaemia and ketosis. It is a medical emergency which if untreated leads to coma and death

Clinical features
1. Gradual onset of weakness and drowsiness over several days, often precipitated by infection, injury or lack of insulin
2. Polyuria, polydipsia and dehydration
3. Deep breathing ('air hunger'), with smell of acetone on the breath
4. Anorexia, abdominal pain and vomiting

Treatment

Principles:
1. Treat the precipitating cause e.g. infection
2. Correct the dehydration and restore the electrolyte balance
3. Re-establish the normal blood sugar level

No inflexible rules can be given but most patients in diabetic coma or pre-coma require 40 to 120 units of soluble insulin (half i.v. and half i.m.) initially, and a saline infusion. Blood is taken immediately for glucose, urea and electrolytes and further treatment depends on the results, with subsequent blood tests at frequent intervals. Hypoglycaemia and hypokalaemia are likely to occur during the recovery stage unless prevented by the infusion of glucose and potassium

HYPOGLYCAEMIC COMA

Due to decreased blood glucose (usually below 40 mg%). Usually precipitated by exercise, a missed meal or insulin overdosage

Clinical features
1. Rapid onset of anxiety, hunger, headache, irritability or unusual behaviour which may progress to coma within a few minutes
2. Rapid bounding pulse, fine tremor, dilated pupils, pallor and sweating
3. Epilepsy may occur, and severe or recurrent hypoglycaemia can cause irreversible cerebral changes or even death

Treatment

Give glucose immediately, by mouth if the patient will co-operate, but failing that, restrain the patient and give 20 ml of 50 per cent dextrose intravenously. Glucagon injection (0.5 to 1 mg subcutaneously) is a suitable alternative

Management of diabetic patients

Life-long careful control of the diabetes is required to postpone complications. The urine must be tested regularly and kept as sugar-free as possible

There are two main types:

1. Juvenile diabetes

Thin young patients who need subcutaneous insulin injections at least once daily. Their physical exercise and diet should be as regular as possible to allow good control to be achieved. Such patients must be taught:

- *i* The importance of good control and how to achieve it
- *ii* How and when to test their urine
- *iii* The techniques of subcutaneous injection, sterilization, insulin dosages etc.
- *iv* The estimation of meal portions according to their dietary allowance
- *v* How to recognize and avert hypoglycaemia
- *vi* The importance of personal hygiene, care of the feet etc.

Insulin injections

These are three main types:

- *i* Rapidly acting but of short duration (6 to 8 hours) e.g. *Soluble insulin*
- *ii* Intermediate e.g. *Insulin zinc suspension* (Lente insulin)
- *iii* Slow but prolonged action (over 24 hours) e.g. *Protamine zinc insulin*

2. Maturity-onset diabetes

Older obese patients who need to reduce to their ideal weight. They can then be controlled on a low carbohydrate diet (e.g. 150 g daily), with the addition of oral hypoglycaemic drugs if necessary

Oral hypoglycaemic drugs

i Sulphonylureas

These act by stimulating the release of insulin from the pancreas e.g. tolbutamide (Rastinon) and chlorpropamide (Diabinese)

ii Biguanides

These augment the action of insulin e.g. phenformin and metformin

Haematology

COMPOSITION OF BLOOD

Blood consists of three 'formed elements' suspended in plasma:
1. *Erythrocytes* (red cells), approx. 5 million/cu.mm
2. *Leucocytes* (white cells), approx. 4 to 10 thousand/cu.mm
3. *Thrombocytes* (platelets), approx. 250 thousand/cu.mm

Haemoglobin, which reversibly binds oxygen, is contained in the red cells in a concentration of about 14g/100 ml of blood

Plasma is a yellow fluid which contains three groups of plasma proteins:
1. *Albumins,* which by their osmotic activity help to control the passage of water from plasma to tissue fluids
2. *Globulins* which constitute the antibody defences against infection
3. *Fibrinogen* and *prothrombin* which are concerned in blood coagulation (p. 100)

The *total blood volume* of an adult is about 4 litres. Of this, plasma occupies 55%, red and white cells occupy 45%, platelets occupy an insignificant volume

FUNCTIONS OF BLOOD

1. **Transport**
    i *Oxygen* from lungs to tissues, and *carbon dioxide* from tissues to lungs
    ii *Products of digestion* from intestines to tissues
    iii *Products of metabolism* from tissues to liver and kidney
    iv *Hormones* from endocrine organs to tissues
2. **Defence against infection**
    i *Humoral.* The immunoglobulins act as antibodies against infectious microorganisms
    ii *Cellular.* The lymphocytes and neutrophils act together to kill bacteria
3. **Coagulation**

RED CELLS

FORMATION OF RED CELLS

Red cells are formed in the bone marrow from nucleated precursor cells called *erythroblasts*. The nucleus disappears before the cells enter the circulation. The newly released red cells, which have a blue-staining reticulum, are called *reticulocytes*. Normally less than 1 per cent of an adult's red cells are reticulocytes but the proportion increases with increased bone marrow activity e.g. after haemorrhage or increased haemolysis

Substances required for the formation and maturation of red cells:

1. *Iron*
2. *Folic acid*
3. *Cyanocobalamin* (vitamin B_{12})

These are present in adequate amounts in a normal mixed diet, but deficiency of one or more may occur if:

1. Diet is abnormal e.g. old people living on bread and jam
2. Malabsorption is present e.g. after gastrectomy
3. Requirements increase e.g. during pregnancy

ANAEMIA

This is a reduction in the amount of haemoglobin in the blood

In *normochromic* anaemia the Hb conc. in each red cell is normal but the total number of cells is decreased

In *hypochromic* anaemia the Hb conc. in each red cell is decreased

Clinical features of anaemia

Symptoms

Tiredness, dyspnoea on exertion, palpitation, giddiness

Signs

1. Pallor of skin, mucosae and conjunctivae
2. Tachycardia
3. Mild ankle oedema

Causes of anaemia

1. *Deficient red cell production*
    - *i* Deficiency of iron, folic acid or cyanocobalamin (vitamin B_{12})
    - *ii* Aplastic anaemia (p. 98)
    - *iii* Marrow replacement with malignant cells
        - Leukaemia
        - Lymphoma (e.g. Hodgkin's)
        - Metastatic carcinoma
    - *iv* 'Symptomatic', i.e. secondary to serious illness
        - Chronic infection
        - Uraemia
        - Rheumatoid arthritis
        - Primary carcinoma

2. *Loss or destruction of red cells*
    - *i* Haemorrhage
    - *ii* Increased haemolysis (p. 99)

IRON DEFICIENCY

This results in the production of small red cells (*microcytes*) which are hypochromic

Common causes

1. Dietary deficiency, especially in elderly
2. Bleeding e.g. from intestinal tract
3. Pregnancy

Treatment

Replacement of iron stones by *ferrous sulphate,* 200 mg b.d. with meals. This may cause gastro-intestinal symptoms and *ferrous gluconate* may be better tolerated. *Iron dextran injection* (Imferon) may be given intramuscularly if oral iron is ineffective, but it may stain the skin, and can cause a generalized reaction

FOLIC ACID AND CYANOCOBALAMIN DEFICIENCY

These result in the production of abnormally large erythroblasts in the marrow (*megaloblasts*). These in turn produce large red cells (*macrocytes*) but the total number of red cells is reduced

Common causes of folate deficiency
1. Poor diet, especially lack of vegetables
2. Malabsorption e.g. coeliac disease
3. Pregnancy

Common causes of cyanocobalamin deficiency
1. Pernicious anaemia (q.v.)
2. 'Blind-loop' syndrome following gastric surgery

PERNICIOUS ANAEMIA

Cyanocobalamin is absorbed from the terminal ileum, but only in the presence of *intrinsic factor* secreted by the gastric mucosa. In pernicious anaemia the gastric mucosa becomes atrophic and fails to secrete intrinsic factor

Clinical features
1. Insidious onset of severe macrocytic anaemia in middle age
2. Skin has a yellowish tinge, often with glossitis (sore tongue)
3. *'Subacute combined degeneration'*:
   B_{12} deficiency can cause degeneration of the peripheral nerves and the posterior and lateral columns of the spinal cord. This produces numbness and tingling of the feet, weakness of the legs and ataxia (inco-ordination). Occasionally these changes develop before the anaemia

Treatment

Large doses of B_{12}, followed by life-long maintenance with hydroxocobalamin (Neo-cytamen) injections (1000 μg i.m. every two months)

APLASTIC ANAEMIA

The red cells, white cells and platelets are greatly decreased due to marrow failure. Such patients often die from infection or haemorrhage

Causes
1. Toxins e.g. benzene
2. Drug reactions e.g. chloramphenicol
3. Many cases are idiopathic

Treatment
1. Isolation from infection
2. Repeated blood transfusion
3. Treatment of infection with antibiotics
4. Steroids to boost the marrow output

HAEMORRHAGE

Anaemia may follow a single massive bleed e.g. severed artery, or the repeated loss of small quantities e.g. peptic ulcer or haemorrhoids. The loss of one pint in an adult produces few symptoms, but the rapid loss of two pints is potentially dangerous. Older people tolerate haemorrhage less well.

Treatment
1. Stop the bleeding if possible
2. Give iron (tablets or injection), blood transfusion or i.v. dextran depending on the severity of the bleeding
3. Morphine is useful for restless patients with severe bleeding

HAEMOLYSIS

Excessive breakdown of red cells in the circulation causes anaemia with an increase in serum bilirubin and urinary urobilin. The increased production of red cells by the marrow produces an increased reticulocyte count (reticulocytosis)

Causes

Congenital
1. Congenital abnormality of red cell (e.g. spherocytosis) or Hb molecule (e.g. sickle-cell anaemia)
2. Haemolytic disease of the newborn, due to rhesus antibodies crossing the placenta in an Rh −ve mother with an Rh +ve baby Antibody formation is prevented by giving mothers at risk an injection of the same antibody (anti-D gamma globulin) within 48 hours of delivery of the first baby

Acquired
1. Poisons (e.g. lead) or infections (e.g. septicaemia, malaria)
2. Antibody formation, idiopathic or secondary to disease (e.g. lymphatic leukaemia)

Treatment of haemolysis

Varies with the cause. Splenectomy or prednisone may help

POLYCYTHAEMIA

Overproduction of red cells by the marrow. The patient looks plethoric and cyanosed due to the increase in circulating red cells. Occasionally white cells and platelets are also produced in excess and a few patients develop leukaemia

BLOOD COAGULATION

Thromboplastin (produced by tissue damage), *platelets* and the other *clotting factors* interact in a complex chain of reactions (the *'coagulation cascade'*) which amplifies the products at each step:

$$\begin{array}{c}\text{Tissue damage}\\\downarrow\\\text{'Coagulation cascade'}\\\downarrow\\\text{Prothrombin}\rightarrow\text{Thrombin}\\\downarrow\\\text{Fibrinogen}\rightarrow\text{Fibrin}\\\downarrow\quad\leftarrow\text{Platelets}\\\text{Blood clot}\end{array}$$

BLOOD TRANSFUSION

Blood groups

There are four main types, A, B, AB and O

In addition, in Britain about 85 per cent of people have the rhesus factor (Rh positive) whereas the remaining 15 per cent are Rh negative

Blood for transfusion must be obtained from a donor of the appropriate ABO blood-group and Rh factor. The donor's cells must be cross-matched with the recipient's serum before use, but in dire emergency a patient may be given group O, Rh negative blood without cross-matching

Complications of blood transfusion

1. Febrile reactions
2. Cardiac failure due to circulatory overload
3. Haemolysis due to blood group incompatibility
4. Thrombophlebitis of the vein
5. Air embolism
6. Transmission of disease from an infected donor (e.g. syphilis, malaria or serum hepatitis)
7. Infected drip site, septicaemia etc. from bacterial contamination of infusion set

BLEEDING DISEASES

May be due to defects in platelets, coagulation factors or vessel wall Spontaneous bleeding into the skin may produce *petechiae* (small purpuric spots) or *ecchymoses* (bruises)

1. **Thrombocytopaenia** (decreased platelet count)

    Causes
    - *i* Idiopathic thrombocytopaenic purpura
    - *ii* Aplastic anaemia (p. 98)
    - *iii* Acute leukaemia (p. 103)

2. **Coagulation defect** (deficiency of a clotting factor)

    Causes
    - *i* Congenital e.g. haemophilia
    - *ii* Acquired e.g. liver disease or anticoagulant drugs

3. **Defects of vessel walls**

    Causes
    - *i* Septicaemia, especially meningococcal
    - *ii* Scurvy (Vitamin C deficiency)
    - *iii* Steroid therapy or Cushing's disease (p. 90)
    - *iv* Vasculitis e.g. Henoch-Schonlein purpura

HAEMOPHILIA

An inherited deficiency of anti-haemophilic globulin (Factor 8). Only males are affected clinically, but females can transmit the disease to their sons. The defect produces prolonged bleeding from minor trauma such as tooth extraction. Bleeding into joints can produce crippling deformity

Treatment

1. Transfusion of fresh blood or Factor 8
2. Splinting of the affected joints

WHITE CELLS
FORMATION OF WHITE CELLS
In a healthy adult about 70 per cent of the circulating white cells are *granulocytes* and 30 per cent are *lymphocytes*

1. **Granulocytes ('polymorphs')**

These are formed in the marrow from precursor cells called *myeloblasts*. As the cells mature they acquire granules in their cytoplasm and their nuclei become irregularly lobed. The mature cells released into the circulation are therefore called *polymorphonuclear granulocytes*

These 'polymorphs' can be subdivided into *neutrophils, eosinophils* and *basophils* according to the staining reactions of their granules. The neutrophils are by far the commonest and they eventually form the *macrophages* which kill and ingest bacteria

2. **Lymphocytes**

These are formed from precursor cells called *lymphoblasts* in the lymphoid tissue (thymus, lymph nodes, marrow and spleen). Lymphocytes are readily distinguished from 'polymorphs' by their dense circular nuclei and scanty cytoplasm

FUNCTIONS OF WHITE CELLS
The granulocytes and lymphocytes co-operate with each other to defend the body against infection. There are two types of lymphocytes (T and B) which look alike but have different functions. Some of the B lymphocytes turn into *plasma cells* which manufacture *immunoglobulins* (antibodies), and the T lymphocytes co-operate with the 'polymorphs' to kill bacteria

All types of white cell appear to be involved in producing the changes of inflammation

LEUCOCYTOSIS
A white cell count exceeding 10 000/cu. mm

Common causes
1. Bacterial infection
2. Haemorrhage or tissue damage (e.g. burns)
3. Leukaemia
4. Malignancy

LEUKAEMIA

A neoplastic disorder of the white cell precursors. It is characterized by immature or abnormal white cells in the blood, and there is usually a marked leucocytosis. Anaemia or thrombocytopaenia may occur due to crowding out of the red cells or platelets by the white cell precursors, and infection is common, since the immature white cells do not function normally

There are two main types:

1. **Myeloid leukaemia**—due to proliferation of granulocyte precursors in the marrow
2. **Lymphatic leukaemia**—due to proliferation of lymphocytes in the lymphoid tissues

Both these diseases may be *acute* or *chronic*

Clinical features of acute leukaemia

1. Fever, malaise, weight loss, anaemia
2. Stomatitis, pharyngitis
3. Susceptibility to infections
4. Bleeding tendency

Acute leukaemia occurs at all ages but is common in young children, and if untreated is rapidly fatal

Clinical features of chronic leukaemia

The symptoms are milder and more insidious than those of acute leukaemia, and the patients are often elderly

In chronic *myeloid* leukaemia the liver and spleen may be greatly enlarged

In chronic *lymphatic* leukaemia the lymph glands are enlarged

Treatment of leukaemia

1. Various combinations of steroids and cytotoxic drugs such as cyclophosphamide or busulphan
2. Blood transfusions as necessary
3. Antibiotics for bacterial infections
4. Irradiation or radio-active phosphorus

LEUCOPAENIA

A white cell count below 4000/cu.mm

Causes

1. Aplastic anaemia
2. Hypersensitivity reaction to a drug e.g. thiouracil

THE LYMPHATIC SYSTEM

The lymphatic vessels convey fluid from the tissues to the lymph glands, and thence to the thoracic lymphatic ducts which drain into the innominate vein in the chest

Causes of lymphadenopathy (enlarged lymph nodes)
1. Infections e.g. skin sepsis, infectious mononucleosis (q.v.)
2. Lymphoma e.g. Hodgkin's disease
3. Lymphatic leukaemia
4. Metastatic carcinoma

INFECTIOUS MONONUCLEOSIS (GLANDULAR FEVER)

An acute infection, probably viral, usually seen in young adults

Clinical features
1. Fever, lassitude, malaise, sore throat
2. Lymphadenopathy and splenomegaly (enlarged spleen)
3. May be a rash
4. Debility and depression which can persist for up to six months

The blood film reveals an excess of lymphocytes, many of which look abnormal. Diagnosis may be confirmed by a Paul-Bunnell agglutination test

Treatment

None, but prolonged convalescence is often necessary

LYMPHOMAS (RETICULOSES)

A group of diseases of varying degrees of malignancy which arise from the lymphoid tissue (the reticuloendothelial system), but which do not produce true leukaemia with abnormal cells in the circulation. Examples of malignant lymphoma include Hodgkin's disease, lymphosarcoma and myelomatosis

Hodgkin's disease

Clinical features
1. Usually young adults
2. Insidious onset of fever, malaise, weakness and anaemia
3. Enlargement of one or more groups of lymph glands
4. Progressively downhill course over several years

Treatment
Deep X-ray therapy or cytotoxic drugs e.g. cyclophosphamide

Myelomatosis

A neoplastic proliferation of plasma cells in the marrow which produce high concentrations of an abnormal immunoglobulin in the blood. This may be excreted in the urine as Bence-Jones protein. Anaemia, bone fractures and renal failure are common

Treatment
1. Cytotoxic drugs e.g. melphelan
2. Blood transfusion as necessary

THE SPLEEN

Functions
1. Blood cell formation
    i   In the *fetus*—red cells and white cells
    ii In the *adult*—lymphocytes
2. Destruction of 'worn-out' red cells and platelets
3. Part of the reticulo-endothelial defence mechanism against infection

Despite these important functions the spleen is not essential for life, and splenectomy is beneficial for some blood disease e.g. spherocytosis

Common causes of splenomegaly (enlarged spleen)
1. Infections e.g. infectious mononucleosis
2. Many blood diseases, especially chronic myeloid leukaemia
3. Portal hypertension

Dermatology

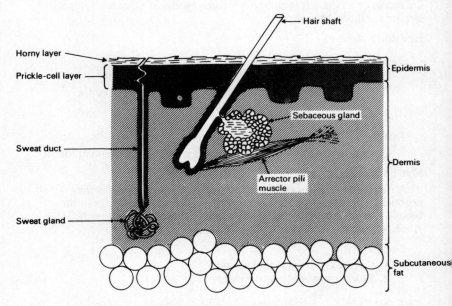

Cross-section of normal skin

    The dermis consists of a dense mat of interweaving collagen bundles permeated by nerves and blood-vessels

FUNCTIONS OF SKIN

1. Retention of tissue fluids and protection of underlying tissues from mechanical damage and infection
2. Regulation of body temperature
   - *i*   Vasoconstriction to conserve heat
   - *ii* Vasodilation and sweating to lose heat
3. Sensory perception
4. Synthesis of vitamin D (p. 112)
5. Psychosexual functions—smooth skin, attractive hair, blushing, etc.

BACTERIAL INFECTIONS

1. Furuncle (Boil)

A deep abscess of a hair follicle due to *Staphylococcus aureus*. Precipitating factors include diabetes and ill-health, but often boils recur for no apparent reason. Such patients are often Staphylococcal 'carriers' and antiseptic nasal cream (e.g. 'Naseptin') and daily chlorhexidine baths may eradicate the bacteria. A *carbuncle* is a larger abscess which discharges pus through several openings. Carbuncles are treated with incision and a systemic antibiotic (e.g. flucloxacillin)

2. Impetigo

A superficial skin infection due to *Staphylococcus aureus*, sometimes with Streptococci in addition. The crusted lesions, which spread readily, are very contagious. Impetigo is sometimes secondary to scabies or pediculosis. Treatment is with antibiotic ointment (e.g. neomycin and bacitracin) but occasionally systemic antibiotics are required

3. Erysipelas

A superficial infection due to *Streptococcus pyogenes* which produces a sharply marginated, red, tender, oedematous area, usually with fever and malaise. *Cellulitis* is a deeper Streptococcal infection which involves the subcutaneous tissues, usually as a complication of a wound or ulcer

Treatment is with intramuscular benzylpenicillin

VIRAL INFECTIONS

1. Verruca (Common wart)

Usually occurs on the hands, or the soles of the feet (plantar wart), but it can also affect the genital and perianal area. Treatments include salicylic acid ointment, podophyllin, freezing, currettage and cautery

2. Herpes simplex ('Cold sore')

Recurrent attacks of localized painful erythema with a group of vesicles (small blisters), usually on the lip. Attacks may be precipitated by a febrile illness or sunshine. Treatment is with an antiviral agent called 5IDU (iododeoxyuridine) applied topically

3. Herpes zoster ('Shingles')

Erythema and grouped vesicles occur in the distribution of a nerve root, due to invasion of a sensory nerve ganglion by the *varicella* (chicken pox) virus. The eruption is often preceded by pain for about two days. Common sites are the chest and face (a branch of the trigeminal nerve)

The rash clears in two to three weeks but severe pain may persist for much longer as *post-herpetic neuralgia*

FUNGAL INFECTIONS

1. Tinea ('Ringworm')

An irritable red scaly rash which tends to clear centrally. The name varies according to the part affected by the fungus:

Tinea *capitis*	— scalp (causes bald patches)
Tinea *corporis*	— face, trunk and limbs
Tinea *cruris*	— inner thighs and scrotum
Tinea *pedis*	— feet ('athletes foot')
Tinea *unguium*	— nails (thickened and discoloured)

Treatment is with fungicidal ointment (e.g. tolnaftate) and if necessary griseofulvin by mouth

2. Candidiasis ('Thrush')

Due to a yeast (*Candida albicans*) which may occur normally in the bowel, but may infect the skin and oral or vaginal mucosa. It produces red patches on the skin, white patches in the mouth and a discharge from the vagina

Predisposing factors:

- *i* Moist, warm skin (e.g. body folds in fat females)
- *ii* Wearing dentures
- *iii* Diabetes or serious illness
- *iv* Systemic antibiotics or steroids
- *v* Pregnancy and oral contraceptives predispose to vaginal candidiasis

Treatment is with Nystatin Ointment, Tablets or Pessaries. The preparation used varies with the site

SKIN PARASITES

1. Scabies

A mite (*acarus*) infestation which causes intense itching. This is due to an allergic reaction to the female mite, which burrows into the epidermis

Treatment is by bathing and then painting the whole body from the neck down with gamma benzene hexachloride (Lorexane) on two successive evenings. Close contacts should also be treated

2. Lice

Three species (head, body and pubic) can infest man. Their eggs may be seen as small white oval bodies (*nits*) attached to the hair or the seams of clothing

Treatment is by gamma benzene hexachloride or DDT, and nits are then removed with a fine-toothed metal comb

3. Fleas and bed-bugs

These insects bite and cause a small irritable wheal (*papular urticaria*)

Treatment is with DDT powder

Dermatology

ECZEMA (DERMATITIS)

A distinctive inflammation of the skin in which the prickle cells of the epidermis become separated by oedema fluid. Clinically there is itching, erythema, papules, vesicles and a variable degree of scaling and weeping

Types of eczema

1. *Exogenous*—due to an external cause
    - *i* Primary irritant dermatitis e.g. caustics, detergents
    - *ii* Allergic contact dermatitis e.g. hypersensitivity to nickel, rubber, dyes etc.
2. *Endogenous*—due to an internal or unknown cause
    - *i* Atopic ('infantile eczema')
    - *ii* Seborrhoeic dermatitis, usually with a very scaly scalp
    - *iii* Varicose eczema of the legs, due to venous stasis

Treatment

If possible the cause is identified and eliminated. Weeping eczema requires an antiseptic bland lotion such as potassium permanganate
Chronic dry eczema requires a steroid or a tar preparation
Sedatives and antihistamines may help to prevent scratching

PSORIASIS

A common inflammatory skin disease with clearly demarcated patches of red skin covered with thick white scales. The cause is unknown, but the basic abnormality appears to be an increased rate of epidermal regeneration in the affected skin. Some patients develop arthritis and nail changes. Psoriasis is sometimes precipitated by Streptococcal tonsillitis

Treatment

1. Topical steroid or tar preparations are useful
2. In severe cases, Dithranol in Lassar's paste is used in combination with a daily tar bath followed by UV irradiation

ACNE VULGARIS

A common disease of adolescence characterized by seborrhoea (greasy skin), comedones (blackheads), papules and pustules. The cause is unknown but blockage of the sebaceous duct and infection with bacteria may be important

Treatment

1. UV irradiation and a variety of topical applications such as retinoic acid (Retin-A) lotion may help
2. A prolonged course of oxytetracycline in low dosage (250 mg daily or b.d.)

ROSACEA

A disease of middle age characterized by redness, papules and pustules of the face, with a tendency to facial flushing and telangiectasia (dilated capillaries). The cause is unknown but the condition is exacerbated by sunlight and heat

Treatment
1. Topical sulphur or hydrocortisone cream may help. Fluorinated steroids (p. 124) should *not* be used
2. A prolonged course of oxytetracycline in low dosage

URTICARIA

Transient wheals with erythema and itching due to histamine release. *Acute* urticaria is often a hypersensitivity reaction to a particular food or drug but the cause of *chronic* urticaria is unknown. Treatment is with oral antihistamines

Angio-oedema is a similar process to urticaria which affects the subcutaneous tissues and the mucous membranes of the mouth and throat. Tracheostomy may be needed if laryngeal obstruction develops

ERYTHEMA NODOSUM

Painful red swellings on the shins which fade to a red-blue colour over two or three weeks. This condition may be precipitated by drugs and infections e.g. TB

ERYTHRODERMA (Exfoliative dermatitis)

Inflammation of virtually the entire skin, followed by desquamation ('peeling'). There is often axillary and inguinal lymphadenopathy, fever and cardiac failure

Causes
1. Widespread eczema or psoriasis
2. Drug rash

DRUG RASH

Virtually any drug can provoke a rash, and virtually any skin disease can occasionally be mimicked by a drug rash

Common causes
1. Antibiotics
2. Barbiturates
3. Sulphonamides

Common types
1. Urticaria
2. Morbilliform (blotchy, like measles)

Drug hypersensitivity often causes pyrexia, and if the drug is not stopped renal or hepatic failure may develop

ANAPHYLACTIC SHOCK

A potentially fatal systemic reaction which may occur if a drug is injected into a sensitized patient. Massive histamine release causes rapid onset of urticaria, angio-oedema, bronchoconstriction and 'shock'. Treatment is with subcutaneous adrenaline and intravenous hydrocortisone and fluid infusion

LEG ULCERS

Causes
1. Stasis ulcers ('Varicose' ulcers)
2. Ulcers due to arterial occlusion or neuropathy

Stasis ulcers

These are secondary to chronic venous stasis due to varicose veins or previous deep vein thrombosis. They occur above the ankle in middle-aged patients and are often surrounded by varicose eczema and pigmentation

Factors which delay healing
1. Anaemia
2. Bacterial infection of the ulcer
3. Lack of adequate supportive dressing
4. Sensitization to a topically applied medicament e.g. an antibiotic or lanolin

Treatment of stasis ulcers
1. Elevation of the leg followed by a firm pressure bandage. Initially this is changed daily but later a paste bandage may be applied for a week or more at a time
2. Treatment of anaemia or bacterial infection
3. Skin grafting may speed healing in suitable cases

Bones and joints

Bone consists of a collagen *matrix* on which are deposited *calcium salts*. It is continually being formed by cells called *osteoblasts* and removed by other cells called *osteoclasts,* so that changes in the shape of a bone ('*re-modelling*') are possible according to the stresses and strains imposed on it. When a patient is confined to bed, these stresses decrease and bone tends to be reabsorbed, with consequent loss of calcium in the urine

RICKETS AND OSTEOMALACIA

Vitamin D (calciferol) increases calcium absorption from the intestine. It is present in milk, butter and eggs and is also formed in the skin by the action of sunlight on a compound derived from cholesterol

Deficiency of vitamin D causes failure of bone calcification, which is called *rickets* in children and *osteomalacia* in adults

Causes of vitamin D deficiency
1. Inadequate diet, especially during pregnancy
2. Malabsorption
3. Lack of exposure to sunlight may aggravate a dietary deficiency

Clinical features of rickets
1. Usually an irritable, sweating, flabby infant with a 'pot-belly'. Failure to thrive is common
2. Bone deformities:
    i Swelling and tenderness of the ends of long bones
    ii Bending of bone may produce bow-legs, scoliosis, pigeon-chest and a narrow pelvis
    iii The skull becomes cuboid and soft
3. Dentition is delayed and the teeth decay easily

Clinical features of osteomalacia
1. Tiredness, weakness and bone pains
2. Minor stresses may cause fractures
3. In severe cases muscle weakness causes a waddling gait

Treatment of rickets and osteomalacia
Daily vitamin D with calcium supplements

OSTEOPOROSIS

An atrophy of bone which affects both calcium and the matrix so that the bone becomes less dense

Causes
1. Old age, possibly related to deficiency of oestrogen or androgen
2. Prolonged immobilization
3. Cushing's disease, or glucocorticoid therapy (e.g. prednisone)

Clinical features
1. May be symptomless, or there may be skeletal pains
2. Loss of height is common, due to vertebral compression, and vertebrae may 'collapse'

Treatment
1. Hormones (androgen, oestrogen or anabolic steroids)
2. Calcium supplements

OSTEITIS DEFORMANS (PAGET'S DISEASE)

A defect in bone re-modelling, with excessive formation of new bone with an abnormal texture. The cause is unknown

Clinical features
1. Middle-aged or elderly patients with pain in the bone
2. Enlarged skull, kyphosis and the tibiae become thickened and curved anteriorly ('sabre-shin')
3. Increased blood flow through the bones may cause cardiac failure

Treatment
Calcitonin infusions

JOINTS

There are three basic types
1. **Fibrous** where no movement is required e.g. skull sutures

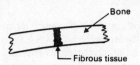

2. **Cartilaginous,** where limited movement is required e.g. pubic symphysis

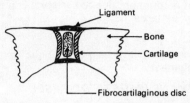

3. **Synovial,** where full movement is required e.g. shoulder, elbow, finger, etc.

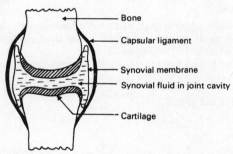

The term *arthropathy* means joint disease. This may be either inflammatory (arthritis) or degenerative

The term *collagen-vascular disease* is applied to a group of overlapping diseases of unknown aetiology which are characterized by the development of auto-antibodies directed against various tissues in the body. The group includes:
1. Rheumatic fever (p. 10)
2. Rheumatoid disease (p. 115)
3. Systemic lupus erythematosus (p. 116)
4. Polyarteritis nodosa (p. 116)
5. Ankylosing spondylitis (p. 116)
6. Dermatomyositis (p. 116)
7. Systemic sclerosis (p. 116)

RHEUMATOID DISEASE

There is no specific diagnostic test for rheumatoid arthritis but in most cases an abnormal globulin (the *rheumatoid factor*) is present in the blood. This is detected by the Rose-Waaler (latex fixation) test

Clinical features
1. Usually affects women in middle life (25–50 yr)
2. Presents as malaise, weight loss, sweating, tachycardia and pain and stiffness in the limbs
3. 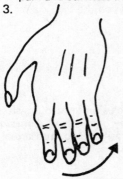 The arthritis usually begins in the small joints of the fingers and wrists and spreads to the ankles, knees and elbows. The joints become hot, swollen and tender. This stage is followed by muscle wasting and characteristic deformities such as *ulnar deviation* of the fingers
4. Associated features may include subcutaneous nodules, anaemia, vasculitis, ocular inflammation and neuropathy

Treatment
1. Rest, with splinting of the joints in the acute stages. Careful attention to posture is necessary and daily physiotherapy is required to avoid joint fixation and muscle wasting
2. Hydrocortisone may be injected directly into the affected joints
3. Systemic drugs:
    i Aspirin in large doses
    ii Prednisone in small doses
    iii Gold injections
    iv Azathioprine
    v Chloroquine
    vi Phenylbutazone or indomethacin
4. Orthopaedic and manipulative measures (wax baths, etc.)

SYSTEMIC LUPUS ERYTHEMATOSUS (SLE)

In this condition an antibody called the *anti-nuclear factor* is directed against DNA (the genetic protein)

Clinical features
1. Usually young or middle-aged women
2. Fever, weight loss, 'flitting' arthritis
3. Pleurisy, pericarditis
4. Renal failure or nephrotic syndrome
5. Rash, especially in 'butterfly' distribution on the face
6. Anaemia
7. Neuropsychiatric changes

Treatment
Prednisone, azathioprine or chloroquine

POLYARTERITIS NODOSA (PN)

In this disease there is inflammation and occlusion of medium-sized arteries and virtually any organ in the body may be involved. Common features include skin ulcers, neuropathy, renal failure and myocardial and intestinal ischaemia

ANKYLOSING SPONDYLITIS

Arthritis of the sacro-iliac joints and vertebral joints produces a painful stiff back ('poker back'). The disease usually starts in young men and is progressive

DERMATOMYOSITIS

Characteristic rash with patchy inflammatory changes in the muscles. Some cases are secondary to internal carcinoma

SYSTEMIC SCLEROSIS

The skin becomes thick and 'bound down' (scleroderma) with Raynaud's phenomenon and digital ulceration. Systemic changes include pulmonary fibrosis and renal failure

Raynaud's phenomenon is transient pallor and cyanosis of the digits due to arterial spasm. It is seen in collagen-vascular disease, but can occur in normal young women

OSTEOARTHROSIS (OSTEOARTHRITIS)

A degenerative process affecting the cartilage and adjacent bone of a large joint (e.g. hip or knee) as a result of prolonged 'wear and tear'. Usually only one joint is involved but some women have multiple symmetrical arthritis affecting the terminal finger-joints

Clinical features
1. Pain in the joints, especially after exertion and in damp weather
2. Creaking is heard or felt when the joint is moved
3. May be osteophytes (bony outgrowth) on the dorsum of the terminal finger-joints

Treatment
1. Rest and physiotherapy
2. Aspirin, phenylbutazone or indomethacin
3. In severe cases, orthopaedic measures e.g. walking-calipers, or hip-joint replacement (prosthesis)

GOUT

Recurrent episodes of arthritis due to increased serum uric acid with deposition of urate crystals in the joints. Gout tends to run in families, and it may be precipitated by rich food, alcohol and thiazide diuretics

Clinical features
1. Usually middle-aged males
2. Sudden excruciating pain in a joint with redness and swelling, accompanied by fever, malaise and irritability. The great toe joint (first metatarso-phalangeal) is classically affected. If untreated the attack lasts for 6 or 7 days
3. Urate crystals are deposited as firm lumps on the subcutaneous tissues, tendons and cartilage (especially on the ears)
4. Renal failure may occur due to uric acid stones and pyelonephritis

Treatment

Acute attack
   i   The affected joint must be carefully protected
   ii The duration of the attack may be decreased by phenylbutazone, indomethacin or colchicine

Chronic gout
   i   Patients should avoid alcohol and purine-rich foods such as liver, kidneys and sweetbreads (pancreas). Obese patients should lose weight
   ii Long-term treatment is needed to reduce uric acid in the body, either by decreasing synthesis in the tissues (*Allopurinol*) or by increasing renal excretion (*Probenecid* or *Sulphinpyrazone*)

FIBROSITIS

A vague condition (also called *myalgia* or *non-articular rheumatism*) with localized pain and tenderness in muscles or ligaments. This includes many cases of 'lumbago', painful shoulders and 'stiff neck'. Precipitating causes include exposure to cold, damp and minor trauma

Treatment
1. Rest and physiotherapy (infra-red radiation and massage)
2. Analgesics such as paracetamol
3. Injection of local anaesthetic or hydrocortisone into the 'trigger-spot'

SCIATICA

Pain in sciatic nerve distribution (back of leg) due to pressure on nerve roots. Often precipitated by coughing, straining, etc.

Causes
1. Intervertebral disc prolapse
2. Lumbar spondylosis (bony outgrowths from the vertebrae)

Drugs

DRUGS USED IN HEART FAILURE

1. Digitalis preparations e.g. digoxin

Actions of digoxin
- *i* Increases the force of ventricular contraction
- *ii* Reduces the heart rate
- *iii* Increases cardiac muscle excitability

Dose of digoxin

0.5 mg three times a day for two or three days to saturate the cardiac tissue; then the dose is reduced to 0.25 mg daily or twice daily. Digoxin is absorbed quickly but excreted very slowly

Features of digoxin overdosage
- *i* Anorexia, nausea and vomiting
- *ii* Pulse rate below 60/min
- *iii* Extrasystoles, often with 'coupling' of the beats (p. 4)
- *iv* Other arrhythmias e.g. heart block, atrial tachycardia

Elderly patients are especially sensitive to digitalis preparations
The effects are enhanced by potassium depletion

2. Diuretics

These are used to treat fluid retention due to failure of the heart, liver or kidneys

i **Thiazides** e.g. hydrochlorothiazide (25 to 100 mg daily) and bendrofluazide (2.5 to 10 mg daily). These increase excretion of potassium, sodium and water, and they also have a hypotensive effect

ii **Frusemide** (*Lasix*). More powerful than the thiazides. The usual oral dose is 40 to 200 mg daily, but it can also be injected i.v.

Potassium supplements are necessary with the above diuretics to prevent hypokalaemia. This is usually given orally in a slow-release form such as *Slow-K,* 2 to 6 tabs daily

iii **Spironolactone** (*Aldactone-A*). This antagonizes the action of aldosterone and thus promotes the retention of potassium. It is particularly useful for cirrhosis or the nephrotic syndrome. The dose is 50 to 100 mg a day in divided doses

3. Aminophylline injection (10 ml containing 250 mg)

This may be slowly injected i.v. to relieve the dyspnoea of pulmonary oedema or asthma. Aminophylline suppositories are also available

DRUGS FOR ARRHYTHMIA

The management of cardiac arrhythmia is complex but the following are commonly used:

1. **Lignocaine, procainamide and phenytoin**

   These suppress ventricular extrasystoles e.g. after myocardial infarction. They may be given i.v. or orally

2. **Beta-blockers e.g. propranolol (*Inderal*) and oxprenolol (*Trasicor*)**

   These are used for arrhythmia due to digoxin overdose or thyrotoxicosis, and for angina pectoris and hypertension. Side-effects include cardiac failure, bradycardia and bronchoconstriction

3. **Isoprenaline**

   This is used to increase the heart rate in heart block, and for asthma. It is given sublingually (10 to 20 mg) or as an aerosol inhalation

ANTICOAGULANTS

1. **Heparin** prevents the activation of prothrombin. It is given intravenously in a dose of 10 000 to 12 500 i.u. and acts immediately. The injections are repeated 6 hrly. to keep the clotting time above 15 mins. The effect can be reversed by **protamine**

2. **Warfarin** prevents the synthesis of prothrombin by antagonizing vitamin K. The initial dose is 30 to 50 mg and the daily maintenance dose is 3 to 10 mg depending on the prothrombin-time estimation. The effect can be reversed by vitamin K_1 i.v.

ANTI-EMETICS

Used for nausea and vomiting

1. **Cyclizine** (*Marzine*), 50 mg three times a day
2. **Chlorpromazine** (*Largactil*), 25 to 50 mg three times a day
3. **Metoclopramide** (*Maxolon*), 10 mg three times a day

PURGATIVES (LAXATIVES, APERIENTS)

1. **Bran and methylcellulose** provide bulk for increased peristasis
2. **Liquid paraffin** softens and lubricates the stools
3. **Senna, and phenolphthalein** act by irritating the bowel

Many proprietary remedies exist e.g. *Dulcolax* is useful in pregnancy, and for the elderly

DRUGS TO CONTROL DIARRHOEA

These either increase the viscosity of the gut contents, or delay their passage

1. **Kaolin and morphine mixture**
2. **Chalk and opium mixture**
3. **Codeine phosphate 30 mg twice daily**

ANALGESICS

The dose depends on the clinical situation e.g. diagnosis, age of patient etc.

1. Aspirin (300 mg tabs)
Chiefly for pain from muscles and joints, but also useful for headaches and dysmenorrhoea. It is anti-inflammatory and anti-pyretic (i.e. reduces fever)

Side-effects
i Indigestion. Prolonged use may cause gastric bleeding
ii In some patients aspirin may provoke asthma or urticaria

2. Paracetamol (500 mg tabs)
This does not cause indigestion but overdosage can damage the liver

3. Codeine phosphate (30 mg tabs)
A relatively weak analgesic which also suppresses cough and produces constipation

4. Dihydrocodeine (*DF118*) (30 mg tabs)
A useful drug for moderate pain

5. Pentazocine (*Fortral*) (25 mg tabs or 30 to 60 mg i.m.)
Useful for severe pain but does not produce the mental detachment which morphine does

6. Pethidine (50 mg tabs or 25 to 100 mg by subcut. or i.m. injection)
Weaker than morphine, but less likely to cause nausea and respiratory depression. Used for labour pains

7. Morphine (10 to 20 mg by subcut. or i.m. injection)
Powerful analgesic, also produces sedation and mental detachment Normally given subcutaneously but in circulatory 'shock' i.v. injection is preferable

Side-effects
i Nausea and vomiting
ii Constipation
iii Respiratory depression
iv Readily produces dependence and addiction

Morphine is dangerous in patients with head injury or chronic respiratory disease

8. Diamorphine (heroin) (5 to 10 mg by subcut. or i.m. injection)
More addictive than morphine but causes less nausea and constipation. Useful for terminal cancer

HYPNOTICS, SEDATIVES AND TRANQUILLIZERS

All these drugs may depress the CNS and their effect is potentiated by alcohol. They also tend to be habit-forming

Hypnotics

1. **Nitrazepam** (*Mogadon*)
   In a dose of 5 mg., its effect lasts about eight hours and the patient wakens fresh. Relatively safe in overdosage
2. **Barbiturates** e.g. sodium amylobarbitone
   In the normal dose of 100 to 200 mg they may cause a 'hang-over', and they can interfere with other drugs e.g. anti-coagulants
3. **Chloral hydrate**
   Chloral mixture (5 to 20 ml) is useful for elderly patients

Tranquillizers

1. **Chlordiazepoxide** (*Librium*) and **diazepam** (*Valium*)
   Both are widely used for anxiety and tension
2. **Barbiturates**
   In small doses (e.g. phenobarbitone 50 mg twice daily) they produce sedation
3. **Chlorpromazine** (*Largactil*)
   Widely used for schizophrenia, and to potentiate the effect of analgesics in terminal illness

DRUGS FOR INFECTIONS

1. **Penicillins**

    Used chiefly for Gram-positive organisms such as Staphylococci and Streptococci
    - *i* **Benzylpenicillin injection** is given i.m. for serious infections which require penicillin, usually 300 mg (500 000 U) every 12 hrs
    - *ii* **Procaine penicillin** has a more prolonged effect
    - *iii* **Penicillin V (Phenoxymethylpenicillin)** is used orally, usually 250 mg every 6 hrs
    - *iv* **Flucloxacillin** (*Floxapen*) is unaffected by penicillinase produced by bacteria and is therefore used for 'resistant' staphylococci
    - *v* **Ampicillin** (*Penbritin*). Not as effective as benzylpenicillin against Streptococci but it has a broader spectrum. Useful for respiratory and urinary tract infections

2. **Cephalosporins** e.g. cephaloridine (*Ceporin*)

    Broad spectrum antibiotics, relatively resistant to penicillinase

3. **Streptomycin** (500 mg to 1 g daily by i.m. injection)

    Used for tuberculosis but the organisms become resistant unless it is used with a second drug (p. 31). In high dosage it is toxic to the kidney and the auditory nerve. Nurses should avoid contaminating their skin with streptomycin as it readily produces allergic contact dermatitis

4. **Tetracyclines**

    Broad-spectrum antibiotics (e.g. oxytetracycline) used for chest infections. The usual dose is 250 to 500 mg every 6 hrs

    Side-effects
    - *i* Gastro-intestinal symptoms e.g. diarrhoea
    - *ii* Predispose to Candidiasis (p. 108)
    - *iii* Prevent absorption of iron and antacids
    - *iv* Cause discolouration of teeth during formation in the fetus and young children

5. **Sulphonamides** e.g. **sulphadimidine**, up to 6 g daily in divided doses

    Useful for urinary tract infections, but allergic reactions with fever and a rash are relatively common

    Co-trimoxazole (*Septrin* 1 tab two to four times a day) is a bactericidal combination of a sulphonamide with a blocker of bacterial folic acid metabolism, which has a broader spectrum than sulphonamides alone

6. **Nitrofurantoin** (*Furadantin*) and **Nalidixic acid** (*Negram*)

    Both are used for urinary tract infections, especially those due to Gram-negative bacteria

GLUCOCORTICOIDS ('STEROIDS')

Uses
1. Used systemically in many serious diseases to suppress inflammation and allergic reactions
2. Used in small doses as replacement therapy in hypoadrenalism
3. Used topically to suppress some inflammatory skin diseases e.g. eczema and psoriasis

Commonly used systemic corticosteroids
1. **Hydrocortisone injection** (i.m. or i.v.)
2. **Cortisone** tablets
3. **Pednisone** tablets (5 times as potent as cortisone)
4. **Bethamethasone** tablets (35 times as potent as cortisone)

Side-effects of prolonged 'steroid' therapy
1. *Exaggeration* of the normal actions of steroids
   - *i* Hypertension
   - *ii* Sodium retention and potassium loss
   - *iii* Diabetes mellitus
   - *iv* Osteoporosis
   - *v* Peptic ulceration
   - *vi* Suppression of growth in children
2. *Suppression of tissue reactions*

This allows infections to spread readily and also 'masks' the clinical signs of infection

3. *Adrenal atrophy* due to suppression of ACTH secretion
   Corticotrophin (ACTH) or its synthetic equivalent, **tetracosactrin** (*Synacthen*) may be injected to stimulate the patient's adrenal glands to secrete hydrocortisone. This avoids the danger of adrenal suppression

Commonly used topical corticosteroids
1. **Hydrocortisone cream or ointment**
2. **Fluorinated corticosteroids**

   e.g. bethamathasone valerate (*Betnovate*)
   fluocinolone acetonide (*Synalar*)

Side-effects
- *i* Prolonged use may cause skin atrophy with striae ('stretch marks')
- *ii* If extensive areas are treated enough corticosteroid may be absorbed to give systemic effects
- *iii* May cause spread of fungus infection

CYTOTOXIC AND IMMUNOSUPPRESSANT DRUGS
1. **Mercaptopurine**
2. **Azathioprine** (*Imuran*)
3. **Methotrexate**
4. **Cyclophosphamide** (*Endoxana*)
5. **Vincristine** (*Oncovin*)
6. **Busulphan** (*Myleran*)

These interfere with cell division of both normal and malignant tissues. Their effect is greatest on rapidly dividing cells such as cancer cells and the normal bone marrow, gastro-intestinal tract, liver and skin. They produce leucopaenia, and the dose is regulated according to the blood count

ELECTROLYTE AND WATER REPLACEMENT

Intravenous infusions are used to replace abnormal losses of body fluids and to correct electrolyte depletion. Special care is required in patients with renal or cardiac disease

Sodium chloride, 0.9 per cent (normal saline)

This is used to replace salt and water, and the kidneys will then correct any moderate disturbance of acid-base balance

Dextrose, 5 per cent

This is used to replace water without salt and it will also provide calories

Sodium bicarbonate, 1.4 per cent

This is used to correct metabolic acidosis e.g. in circulatory 'shock' or after cardiac arrest

Addition of medication to i.v. fluids

This is required if intermittent injection is dangerous, as with potassium chloride, or if constant blood levels are required, as with heparin

Latin abbreviations used in prescribing

These are officially frowned upon but nevertheless they continue to be used by many doctors

a.c.	before meals
ad lib.	as much as desired
alt. die	alternate days
alt. nocte	alternate nights
b.d. / b.i.d.	twice daily
c̄	with
ex. aqua	in water
n. et m.	night and morning
o.m.	every morning
o.n.	every night
p.c.	after meals
p.r.n.	repeat as required
q.i.d.	four times daily
q.s.	a sufficient quantity
rep.	to be repeated
s.o.s.	if necessary (a single dose)
stat.	immediately
t.d.s. / t.i.d.	thrice daily

Index

Absorption, 35, 37
Acne vulgaris, 109
Acute nephritis, 75
Adrenal failure, 89
Air hunger, 21
Aminophylline, 119
Anaemia, 95, 96
Analgesics, 121
Anaphylactic shock, 111
Anatomy
    central nervous system, 52
    gastro-intestinal tract, 35
    heart, 1
    liver, 47
    meninges, 57
    renal tract, 67
    reproductive system, 80, 81
    respiratory tract, 19
    spinal cord, 54
Angina pectoris, 14
Ankylosing spondylitis, 116
Anorexia, 39
Antibiotics, 123
Anti-coagulants, 120
Anti-emetics, 120
Aortic stenosis, 12
Aplastic anaemia, 98
Arrhythmia
    classification, 8
    treatment, 120
Ascites, 44
Asthma, 28
Ataxia, 56
Athetosis, 55
Atrial fibrillation, 4
Atrial flutter, 8
Atrial septal defect, 10

Bacterial endocarditis, 12
Bleeding diseases, 101
Blood, 94
Blood pressure, 6
Bone formation, 112
Bradycardia, 3
Bronchial cancer, 32
Bronchiectosis, 27
Bronchitis, 24
Bronchopneumonia, 26

Calculi, 79
Candidiasis, 108
Cardiac
    arrest, 16
    cycle, 2
    output, 1
    failure, 13
Carpal tunnel sydrome, 65
Cellulitis, 107
Central nervous system, 52
Cerebrospinal fluid, 56
Cerebrovascular disease, 62
Chest
    pain, 15
    shape, 22
Cheyne—Stokes breathing, 21
Cholecystitis, 50
Cholelithiasis, 50
Chorea, 10
Choreiform movements, 55
Cirrhosis, 49
Clubbing, 22
Coagulation, 100, 101
Coarctation, 9
'Cold sore', 107
Colic, 43
Collagen vascular disease, 113
Coma, 60
Congenital heart disease, 9
Constipation, 44
Cough, 23
Cranial nerves, 53
Cretinism, 87
Crohn's disease, 45
Cushing's disease, 90
Cyanocobalamin, 97
Cyanosis, 29
Cystitis, 77
Cytotoxic drugs, 125

Deep vein thrombosis, 17
Dermatitis, 109
Dermatomyositis, 116
Diabetes insipidus, 86
Diabetes mellitus, 91
Diabetic ketosis, 92
Diarrhoea
    causes, 43
    treatment, 120

Diastole, 2
Digestion, 35, 36
Digoxin, 119
Disseminated sclerosis, 64
Diuretics, 119
Diverticulitis, 46
Drug rash, 110
Duodenal ulcer, 41
Dyspepsia, 40
Dysphagia, 38
Dyspnoea, 6, 21
Dysuria, 73

Eczema, 109
Electrolytes, 125
Embolism, 18
Emphysema, 25
Entero-hepatic circulation, 48
Epilepsy, 61
Erysipelas, 107
Erythema nodosum, 110
Erythroderma, 110
Exfoliative dermatitis, 110
Extradural haematoma, 62
Extrasystoles, 4

Facial palsy, 53
Faeces, 42
Fallot's tetralogy, 9
Female genitalia, 80
Fibrositis, 118
Flaccidity, 55
Folic acid deficiency, 97
Frequency of micturition, 73
Furuncle, 107

Gastric ulcer, 41
Gastro-enteritis, 45
Gastro-intestinal hormones, 36
General paralysis of the insane, 59
Glomerulonephritis, 75
Glucocorticoids, 89
Glycosuria, 71
Goitre, 86
Gonorrhoea, 82
Gout, 117
Grand mal attack, 61
Granulocytes, 102

Haematemesis, 39
Haematuria, 71
Haemolysis, 99
Haemophilia, 101
Haemorrhage, 98

Heart, 1
Heart block, 8
Hepatitis, 49
Herpes simplex, 107
Herpes zoster, 107
Hiatus hernia, 40
Hodgkin's disease, 105
Hydrocephalus, 56
Hyperparathyroidism, 88
Hyperpituitarism, 85
Hypertension, 7
Hyperthyroidism, 87
Hypnotics, 122
Hypoadrenalism, 90
Hypoglycaemic coma, 92
Hypoparathyroidism, 88
Hypopituitarism, 86
Hypotension, 6
Hypothermia, 34
Hypothyroidism, 87

Impetigo, 107
Incontinence, 72
Incoordination, 56
Industrial lung disease, 27
Infectious mononucleosis, 104
Innocent murmurs, 10
Insect bites, 108
Insomnia, 66
Intestinal obstruction, 44
Intracerebral haemorrhage, 62
Intracranial tumour, 60
Iron deficiency, 96

Jaundice, 48
Joints, types of, 114
Jugular venous pulse, 5

Leg ulcers, 111
Leucocytosis, 102
Leucopaenia, 103
Leukaemia, 103
Lice, 108
Liver, 47
Lobar pneumonia, 25
Lung tumours, 32
Lymphadenopathy, 104
Lymphocytes, 102
Lymphomas, 105

Malabsorption, 42, 43
Male genitalia, 81, 82
Meningitis, 57
Menstrual cycle, 80, 81

Index

Micturition, 72, 73
Migraine, 63
Mineralocorticoids, 89
Mitral incompetence, 12
Mitral stenosis, 11
Motor neurone disease, 64
Motor pathway, 54
Muscle wasting, 65
Muscular dystrophy, 66
Myasthenia gravis, 66
Myelomatosis, 105
Myocardial infarct, 15
Myocardial ischaemia, 14
Myxoedema, 87

Nephron, 67
Nephrotic syndrome, 76
Neuropathy, 65
Neurosyphilis, 59
Non-specific urethritis, 84

Oliguria, 68
Ophthalmoplegia, 53
Optic neuritis, 53
Orthopnoea, 6
Osteitis deformans, 113
Osteoarthritis, 117
Osteomalacia, 112
Osteoporosis, 113
Oxygen therapy, 29

Pacemaker, 2
Paget's disease, 113
Pancreas, 51, 90
Pancreatitis, 51
Paralysis, 55
Paralysis agitans, 63
Parathyroids, 88
Parkinsonism, 63
Paroxysmal tachycardia, 8
Peptic ulcer, 41
Pericarditis, 16
Peripheral neuritis, 65
Peristalsis, 36
Pernicious anaemia, 97
Persistent ductus orteriosus, 9
Petit mal, 61
Phlebitis, 18
Pituitary, 85
Plasma, 94
Pleurisy, 33
Pneumoconiosis, 27
Pneumonia, 25
Pneumothorax, 33

Poliomyelitis, 58
Polyarteritis nodosa, 116
Polycythaemia, 99
Polyuria, 68
Prescribing, 126
Proteinuria, 71
Psoriasis, 109
Pulmonary oedema, 14
Pulmonary stenosis, 9
Pulse, 3—5
Purgatives, 120
Pyelonephritis, 77, 78
Pyrexia, 34

Red cells, 95
Reflexes, 54
Refractory period, 2
Regional ileitis, 45
Reiter's syndrome, 84
Renal
   calculi, 79
   failure, 74, 76
   function, 68
   tract, 67
Renin-angiotensin system, 89
Respiration, 20, 21
Retention of urine, 72
Rheumatic fever, 10
Rheumatic heart disease, 11
Rheumatoid disease, 115
Rickets, 112
Rigor, 34
Ringworm, 108
Rosacea, 110

Scabies, 108
Sciatica, 118
Sensory pathway, 54
Sex hormones, 81, 82, 85, 89
Shingles, 107
Sinus arrhythmia, 4
Skin, 106
Space-occupying lesions, 60
Spasm, 55
Spasticity, 55
Spinal cord, 54
Spleen, 105
Sputum, 23
Status asthmaticus, 28
Status epilepticus, 61
Steroids, 89, 124
Stoke-Adams attacks, 8
Stomach, 38
Stomatitis, 38

Stroke, 62
Subacute combined degeneration, 97
Subarachnoid haemorrhage, 62
Subdural haematoma, 62
Syncope, 60
Syphilis, 12, 83
Syringomyelia, 64
Systemic lupus erythematosus, 116
Systemic sclerosis, 116
Systole, 2

Tabes dorsalis, 59
Tachycardia, 3
Temperature, 34
Tertiary syphilis, 59
Thrombocytopaenia, 101
Thrombosis, 17
'Thrush', 108
Thyroid, 86
Thyrotoxicosis, 87
Tinea, 108
Tongue, 38
Tranquillizers, 122
Transfusion, 100

Tremor, 55
Trichomonas vaginalis, 84
Trigeminal neuralgia, 53
Tuberculosis, 30, 31

Ulcerative colitis, 46
Uraemia, 74
Urine
    colour, 69
    microscopy, 71
    quantity, 68
    specific gravity, 69
    testing, 69–71
Urticaria, 110

Venereal disease, 82–84
Ventilation, 20
Ventricular septal defect, 10
Verruca, 107
Vessel wall defects, 101
Vitamins, 37
Vomiting, 39

White cells, 102

Notes